THE COURAGE TO THINK DIFFERENTLY

A Bold Investigation of Prejudice, Human Behavior, and the Power to Revolutionize the Ideas that Shape Our World

STEVEN H. HARLEM, PH.D.

Publishing Services provided by Paper Raven Books

Printed in the United States of America

First Printing, 2019

Paperback ISBN= 978-1-7327700-0-3
Hardback ISBN= 978-1-7327700-1-0

To those teachers and students who had infinite patience with me while nourishing a passion and need for continual learning.

TABLE OF CONTENTS

PREFACE

My interest in writing this book stems from the painful reality of increasing violence, mental illness, and a variety of other significant social ills in our country. While there are no simple solutions, I believe, after working 45 years in a variety of medical-related and teaching fields, there are better approaches to help remediate much of the unmerited pain and helplessness that currently permeates our society.

To this end, I present historical and personal vignettes that, at times, on the surface may appear unrelated but they share central unifying themes. If we want to better understand and effectively intervene in human actions, there is the necessity of holding alternative models—multiple ways with which to view human behavior. In addition, it may also be necessary to challenge established authorities to better comprehend, for example, suicide, depression, along with other expressions of deviance in both individuals and groups as well as the communication that perpetuates these behaviors. To do this will require courage.

My hope is that you, the reader, whether in a professional field, a student in college or high school, or anyone who delights in the joy of discovery and personal growth, might derive some benefit from the following odyssey.

Introduction

Throw a stone into the water and the ripples can theoretically go on forever. It is not an exaggeration to say individuals do not readily give up their entrenched beliefs even if they are proven wrong. These convictions, like a stone dropped into a pool, spread their ripples with a force and a life that is often far too long that ultimately impedes progress.

The history of mankind is written in steps. Not all are forward. My hope is this book will help you become aware of your beliefs and the models that shape your perceptions, understandings, and habits of questioning human interactions. We often forget that the models to which we subscribe are not synonymous with truth. In fact, they may work against our seeing the truth and even harming those we wished to help. Our goal is to leave ourselves open to holding alternative models. Since our beliefs determine the questions we ask and the answers we receive, we should attempt to develop multiple ways of seeing and questioning—these are our models. This approach permits us to tease out the truths from the myths of our society and more effectively comprehend the complexities of human behavior.

In the broader sense, this book is an appeal to the minds and hearts of the reader to search for the truth. As you read, you will witness obstacles and difficulties, divisions and indifference, and even callousness. As Antoine de Saint-Exupéry writes in *Wind, Sand and Stars,* "We are not separated by our truths but by our passions with which we embrace our truths." Putting aside our passions, we realize that our clothes and our music reflect the influence of our times, so too can our education. This is true in science, in medicine, in mental health, and in laws and punishments, and is reflected in our entrenched beliefs. These convictions are communicated to us, with and without language, within the social system in which we reside. This communication determines those standards than can advance or retard our ways of thinking and behaving. Human history is replete with this lesson. And it is to some of this history we now turn.

Before we do, please keep in mind that those of us who put forth personal or professional opinions have human frailties. All of us are plagued at times by arrogance, personal insecurity, misunderstanding, jealousy, greed, and self-centeredness. These time-honored human failings, in the best of us, foster resistance to consider new ideas. William James cautioned us when he wrote, "The greatest enemy of our truths may be the rest of our truths."

Six thousand years ago, the Chaldean priests mapped the stars. The Greek philosopher

Anaximander suggested the earth floats in space, and the order of the world was due to natural and not supernatural forces. By 3,000 BC, the length of the year had been computed with a deviation of less than .001 percent. Aristarchus, born in 310 BC, put forth the idea that the earth revolves around the sun. After these Greek and Babylonians, whose theories were largely ignored, came the Pythagorean brotherhood with an unsound model of the universe that influenced the world for 17 centuries (32). Remember, it was not only tradition, prejudice, and naïve common sense but also the scientific evidence that spoke later against the more accurate Copernican theory (41). The danger is ever-present today that someone will come up with yet another denial of a scientific fact, such as global warming, and then support it using pseudoscience. Since our beliefs influence what we see and how we act, can there be unbiased evaluations or understanding with biased minds? When it comes to scientific models, always ask whose good is served by that model. There is always the necessity to consider alternative models or ways of viewing life events. This is vividly illustrated in our next example.

In the early part of the 19th century, the practice of physicians was still influenced by the beliefs and techniques employed by the Greek and Roman physicians 2,000 years earlier. Disease was often attributed to fever and inflammation due to overeating. Other diseases diagnosed as phthisis may have been the result of exposure to unwholesome air, grief, playing wind instruments to excess, debaucheries, cold weather, moisture, and so on. Since disease was frequently associated with increased body heat caused by fever and inflammation, the treatment was to reduce the excessive heat. Among the solutions, bloodletting was quite prevalent, making leeches quite popular (11).

While autopsies were performed, it was often to aid in the teaching of anatomy. However, by the end of the 19th century, pathological anatomy began to have a greater influence on medical instruction and thinking. The impetus fueling this change was the discovery of tumors called "tubers" in the lungs of certain patients with phthisis. This "tuberous phthisis" came to be called tuberculosis.

As Carter and Carter point out in *Childbed Fever,* during the early 19th century, charity hospitals, like the Vienna General Hospital, were operating in most of the major cities of Europe. Many of their patients were indigent and treated without payment. Therefore, upon their death, it was considered reasonable they pay for this charity by donating their bodies for dissection. Despite the knowledge gained through dissection, the prevailing view of disease remained largely unchanged. Diseases were caused by atmospheric influences.

Despite the pressures to conform, there have always been those who think and see things differently and more clearly. There were advances in several medical areas. Dr. Joseph Skoda popularized the use of the stethoscope. Dr. Ferdinand Hebra founded modern dermatology, and Dr. Jakob Kolletschka specialized in forensic pathology. Unfortunately, the thinking of these men did not influence the practice of those working in the maternity wards, as the death rate among women remained extremely high.

It was actually safer to deliver your child in the street than in the hospital. Official documents referred to the maternity clinics as houses of death. There were two sections in the maternity clinics. The first, in the mid-1800s, was run by obstetrical students who, before examining their expecting patients, dissected cadavers. The second section was served by female midwives who did not dissect prior to attending to the expecting mothers. The death rate in the first section was much higher than in the second section, but death continued to be attributed primarily to the local miasmas.

When the death rate was especially high—termed childbed fever—walls were cleaned, floors scrubbed, and bloodletting was the treatment of choice. Twenty years later, despite the suffering of these terrified women and countless deaths, nothing changed. The symptoms of childbed fever or "puerperal fever" (meaning a woman who had just given birth) included: acute and intense pain, increased pulse, fever, shortness of breath, shortness of milk, and delirium, to name a few (11).

In 1847, a Hungarian obstetrician, Dr. Ignaz Semmelweis, joined the staff of the Vienna Hospital. He trained in midwifery and was assigned to the first section. He was described as a gentle and sensitive man who was appalled and tormented by the reality of the 20 percent mortality rate from childbed fever. In order to determine a cause for puerperal fever, Semmelweis conducted autopsies like the physicians who preceded him. Following the dissections, he would make his morning rounds in the first section of the maternity clinic, as did the other physicians. Although moved by the begging and pleading of the women to be assigned to the second section, he remained powerless to change the nightmare and outcome of puerperal fever. He was, in certain ways, a product of his time and believed that the usual factors such as inadequate ventilation, problems with a pregnant uterus, excess blood, and stagnation of the circulation were partly responsible for the mortality rates. However, he was unable to explain why the mortality rate was so different between the two sections when the same conditions existed in both.

He eventually learned that his close friend Dr. Jakob Kolletschka had died from symptoms that were identical to childbed fever. Apparently, while conducting a dissection, the professor's finger was stuck by a student with the same instrument used in that autopsy. Semmelweis was the person who looked at the same facts, but thought and saw something different than the other physicians.

Despite washing their hands after an autopsy, the physicians' hands and nails still smelled from the decaying matter. A typical washing simply could not remove the residue. Semmelweis concluded that the students and physicians themselves were transmitting the disease from the dissections directly during the examination of their pregnant patients. He believed that particles from the cadavers were absorbed by the patient during gynecological examinations. This transmission occurred when the physicians' hands came in contact with the exposed uterus or the genital tract lesions caused by the birth process. This meant the doctors themselves caused childbed fever.

Semmelweis found that if the doctors washed their hands with a chlorine solution, the death rate dramatically dropped. He demanded and often had to resort to begging the doctors in his ward to scrub their hands and nails before examining a patient. It has been written that he, at times, would sit in the doorway of the first ward next to the chlorine solution to make sure the attending doctors washed. This solution was quite inexpensive and effective in reducing the mortality from childbed fever to one percent. When new medical students began training in the first section, death rates rose again. However, if the new physicians were forced to wash their hands in the chlorine solution, mortality again dropped. Semmelweis concluded that exposure to any kind of decaying matter might be conveyed in ways other than the hands. These were the days before sterile gloves and white coats, and it was a kind of prestige for a physician to have some cadaveric material remaining on their vest. As Semmelweis's accomplishments spread across Europe, many physicians adopted chlorine washing with the same benefits to their patients. Despite these successes, resentment against Semmelweis increased and he was ultimately dismissed from his position.

The influence of Dr. Semmelweis, saved thousands of lives. Even so, it flew in the face of the prevailing, time-honored, or superstitious dogmas about the etiology of disease. Critics pointed out that doctors and students did wash their hands with soap and water before examinations. "How could contaminants in such infinitesimal amounts possibly cause such damage?" Critics even blamed his theory of infectious particulates on his Catholic faith. Childbed fever was due not to invisible particles, but to Catholic superstition and the presence of priests bearing the Eucharist to frightened dying patients (13).

After his dismissal, Semmelweis instituted chlorine washings at three other hospitals with the same positive outcomes. Yet his idea continued to be ridiculed and often rejected in Vienna and Budapest. How could doctors be responsible for killing their patients? Semmelweis never published the logic behind his theory, though it may not have made a difference. He did, however, rail against the European medical establishment that attacked him. Despite his contributions, he was described as an embarrassment to his medical colleagues and family. In 1865, Semmelweis was committed to a Viennese insane asylum under questionable circumstances. Fifteen days later, after his admission, he died. His autopsy was conducted in the same dissection rooms at the Vienna General Hospital where he himself had performed autopsies. The findings of his autopsy revealed blood poisoning and severe internal injuries resulting from beatings in the asylum (11).

From our perspective, it seems impossible that Semmelweis's claims, and the fact that thousands of lives were saved, could be rejected. One has to understand, at that time, he went against what almost everyone else thought about disease causation. This alienated him from most of the physicians in Europe. It would take another 20 years before Joseph Lister made a more persuasive argument for antisepsis in surgery.

As we will see, times change more rapidly than people. Part of what can be gleaned from the experiences of Semmelweis is that most people are closed to new ideas. Perhaps sensitivity removes the scales from the eyes of some observers, but this does not guarantee an openness to change. Sensitivity often generates hunches and, for some, a new insight. I encourage the reader, should this happen to them, not to hesitate to express their ideas a priori as long as they are taken as such. Ideas can always be modified and even completely transformed by the observation of facts. It is quite exciting and rewarding to view a problem from a different position. Make your view sufficiently public so that others can test and further explore your own findings. By this approach, you communicate your knowledge or perspective instead of expecting others to accept it on faith. I find it difficult to tolerate those who doubt everything as an excuse to do nothing.

Moving forward to the 19th century, it is easy to find examples of this resistance to consider new ideas. Gregor Mendel, an Augustinian friar and scientist, is considered the founder of modern genetics. Between 1856 and 1863, his pea plant experiments established many of the rules of heredity. We now refer to them as the laws of Mendelian inheritance. However, when he presented his research in 1865, he was essentially ignored by the scientific community for the next 35 years (37).

Racism and bigotry, additional expressions of closed minds, are no strangers to the scientific community. A number of years ago, Cyril Burt, a well-respected geneticist, "proved" that Caucasians were genetically superior to blacks. A graduate student was startled to discover he faked his data so that he might arrive at the conclusion he wanted or perhaps needed (6).

Dr. Charles Drew, an exceptional physician whose life was dedicated to saving lives, had to constantly struggle with racial discrimination his entire life. He was an outstanding athlete in high school and college and was named to the all-American team at Amherst College in Massachusetts but, when traveling with the football team to away games, he was denied admittance to restaurants because he was an African American. He ultimately attended medical school at McGill University in Montreal, Canada and eventually took a residency at Columbia University Presbyterian Hospital in New York where he became interested in research on blood and blood transfusions.

Dr. Drew found that while everyone has a certain blood type and could only accept a transfusion from a donor with the same type, we all have the same type of plasma. His discovery led to the battlefield transfusions that saved countless lives of

American soldiers as well as the lives of our injured allies. He was eventually named project director for the American Red Cross but resigned his position after the United States War Department issued a directive that blood taken from white donors should be segregated from that of black donors. He wrote,

"One can say quite truthfully that on the battlefields nobody is very interested in where the plasma comes from when they are hurt.... It is unfortunate that such a worthwhile and scientific bit of work should have been hampered by such stupidity" (16).

There was, around the same time, a professor at Northwestern University who wrote a book proving the Holocaust never happened. During 1924, immigrants from Eastern Europe were given English language IQ tests at Ellis Island in order to set the immigration quota. At that time, if one was feeble-minded, determined by their performance on these IQ tests, they were denied entry into the United States. Dr. Herbert Jennings, a biologist, was quite vocal in his opposition to this absurdity of giving an IQ test in English to those who never spoke the language. Immigration bias continues to impact our society today (27).

Many hold assumptions about the behavior of individuals or groups based upon their race, their accents, religion, and nationality. How many social problems result from people assuming the behavior of the individual is reducible to these kinds of characteristics? The behavior of an individual does not reside, for example, in their color. Race does not define a propensity for a particular behavior. We must examine our own assumptions, our own language, if we are to tease out the myths to which our society and we ourselves often subscribe. Without this self-examination, we allow the causes of prejudice, arrogance, and violence to continue unchecked. Tersely put, the goal is to remove the scales from our eyes and minds. I also believe the desire to achieve, to become better in what we do, while deeply personal, is also embedded in the hearts of most.

Time brings inevitable change, and today we are experiencing an exponential rise in knowledge and evidence that our world in changing. I believe it is easier for a physicist to determine the number of subatomic particles than for individuals to change their ideas and behaviors. If I am correct, this is unfortunate as it cheats not just others but ourselves as well, and we lose the magic inherent in thinking and discovery.

Our universe is measured to be 13.8 billion years old, although there are some who hold alternative truths about this. Inside the atom, our traditional concepts of space and time are no longer valid. How do we make sense of some of these changes that have impacted our lives? One way is simply to become aware of these shifts in thinking.

The great physicist Richard Feynman showed us that a particle, a positron, can move backward in time. The movement of this positron, known as antimatter, insinuates that perhaps today caused yesterday. This can be somewhat disarming when the implication is the past may not completely determine the future. When antimatter slows and hits ordinary matter, they both explode and typically emit gamma rays that are absorbed and turned into heat. Matter-antimatter annihilation is used on a daily basis in hospital PET scans. The P in PET is for the positron that emits certain radioactive chemicals, such as iodine-121.

Without Einstein's theory of relativity, we would not have the GPS devices we now have. Physicists now know that time changes in that it stretches, bends, and may now even be reversible. If our GPS satellites did not take relativity into consideration, they would miss our location by miles. The iPhone has an internal clock that runs 1.4 billion cycles every second. It is amazing this little device, owned by most of us, is dependent upon Einstein's theory of relativity.

It is also interesting to consider that when you fly at the average speed of a commercial airplane, let us say 500 plus miles per hour, you are younger by 29 nanoseconds (billionths of a second a day). If interested in understanding this phenomenon, the reader is encouraged to read about time dilation for a better understanding of the above.

Einstein's theories derived not from traditional experimentation, but through his openness to think about cosmic events differently from the classical physicists. Through his mind experiments, he developed alternative models that he believed explained how the world worked. In doing so, he changed our lives forever. Despite experimental verification, it took time before many scientists of his day could overcome their resistance to give up their time-honored concepts and convictions (38).

It is not uncommon to see scientific theories emerge, prevail for a time, and ultimately vanish. Other theories that initially were rejected often have a way of conquering later generations. Science constantly challenges us to rethink our understanding about the world. Scientists as well as others not only record the facts, but they also often conform to them without questioning, which may not always be conducive to advancement.

As you read through the following chapters, I will present results from the past and present that are surprising, interesting, enlightening, and even challenging. My goal is to sensitize you to the necessity of considering alternative models or ways of viewing life events. The flexibility you cultivate through the ability to work with multiple models and perspectives can make you more effective in your interactions with others as well as enhance your personal and professional growth. Chapters 2, 3, and 4 will review the models and their impact on how we understand human interaction. These include the medical model, the psychological model (psychiatry included), and the sociogenic model. This last model is perhaps the one we are least familiar with but, in my opinion, its importance cannot be overstated. Its emphasis on nonverbal communication determines more of human behavior than is commonly considered. It is, for me, a most exciting model. Still, I prefer to travel among all three models when working with individuals, as no one model can explain all behavior. The thread that is woven through all three models is my belief that you, the reader, will combine your individual experiences with your empathy and intellect to become better at what you do.

CHAPTER 1

Resistance to Change

As you will see in this chapter, the events will be largely personal to a degree, but I will not be wallowing in my own personal wisdom.

I was 27 years old and a junior in college majoring in psychology. At that time, I had an internship in a large state mental hospital and, because I was older than the typical junior, was permitted to work with 44 patients whose primary diagnosis was alcoholism. The hospital was located in Haverford, Pennsylvania in a lovely country setting. There were 21 buildings on the hospital grounds, each serving patients with different diagnoses.

I was responsible for planning a picnic for the hospital residents. One Friday, I took 22 patients from my building to the arts and crafts room located in the administration unit in order to make signs for the upcoming event.

The following Monday, I was called to meet with the hospital administrator. I sat down in his office and he asked me, "Did you give scissors to the patients?" I responded that I had, and asked if any were missing. None were missing and the room had been left in order. His concern was that I allowed patients to use scissors without adequate supervision.

I sincerely apologized and as I left his office, I stopped at the door and said to him, "Did you ever think the reason no scissors were missing is because I did not expect them to be?" When I left him and returned to my building, I was initially filled with a hesitant pride and also frightened. I felt myself ill-prepared for the responsibility the professional staff had placed upon me. It would take me another 10 years to fully understand the comment I had made to the administrator and the professional journey of a lifetime to feel somewhat more secure.

While at this hospital as an undergraduate, I had a clinical psychology internship. The department of psychology at my hospital had at least four Ph.D. psychologists on their staff. I felt the psychology staff was influenced by their training and their subsequent professional experiences. I had a distinct advantage as my thinking was not yet fixed by my limited preparation. This left me free to wander off of a fixed path of thinking and, at that time, I was not concerned about a career track. Between 1964 and 1965, these psychologists were all vying for federal grant money as another hospital, a former tuberculosis sanitarium, was being refurbished and reopened as a new facility to treat alcoholism and drug addiction. In addition to grant funds, the incentives for the psychologists at my hospital included treatment innovations for the above addictive illnesses plus a staff appointment to the new facility.

A 60-year-old gentleman who suffered from chronic alcoholism was selected to be the subject of their treatment. I was given the responsibility to aid in the therapy of this man during the seven-month study.

I was obligated to take the subject to a room where he would watch a slide presentation of various scenes, some of which were associated with alcohol use and others of which were not. The subject had the slide projector control and could change any slide at will. There were also two electrodes attached to the fingers on his right hand. I watched the same scenes through a two-way mirror in an adjacent room where I had the controls to administer a shock. When a scene had something to do with alcohol use, I had to deliver a shock that was terminated as soon as the subject changed the slide from an alcohol-associated scene to one that reflected the benefit of abstaining from alcohol. I should mention the shock to the fingers was not severe but annoying and unpleasant.

I explained to my superiors, one of which was my university department chairman, that I believed several important variables were missing in their experimental design. I felt drinking was not simply a behavior isolated from other environmental variables. There were many other factors associated with drinking including the sights, smells, sounds, feelings, and relationships experienced in bars. I believed that the behaviors associated with alcohol use were quite complex. I attempted to make the treatment more realistic by replicating a drinking environment as much as possible. I asked for permission to bring whiskey into the hospital for the study, and I went to several bars and recorded the sounds of people enjoying their social hour. I played these recordings when the drinking slides were presented on the screen. After several months, I obtained permission to use the whiskey but was only allowed to put exactly seven drops, seven only, in a shot glass and give it to the subject. When he would try, literally, to suck out the whiskey, he was shocked until he put down the glass. What was not disclosed to me was that in addition to the aversive conditioning I was administering, the patient was receiving alternative therapies seven days each week for the seven months. The motivation for the grant money and professional recognition pushed the psychologists to tweak this treatment to facilitate a positive outcome.

The seven months of treatment finally ended on a Friday. The four psychologists responsible for the "cure" were in a jubilant mood. They had arranged for the subject to have a job in Washington, DC beginning the following Monday. I remember sitting silently in the department as I watched the four primary clinicians congratulating themselves. Finally, one of the psychologists, noting my silence, asked me what I thought. I replied, "It won't work." A complete silence fell over the room with no one responding to me, and we all shortly left the hospital.

The next morning, I received an early phone call telling me they had found our subject "dead drunk" on the subway platform. Monday morning, back at the hospital, I was asked, "How did you know what would happen?"

My answer was, "You took away a behavior (i.e., drinking) but what did you give him in return to take its place?" I had come to know the subject reasonably well in the seven months as I watched him struggle with the program. This helped me see things differently from the others. They tried to eliminate a behavior that, for better or for worse, enabled this man to function in his life. I was able to focus on the man himself and not be overly influenced by the experimental outcome that was shaped by other incentives.

After graduation, I next finished my master's degree and was to attend the University of New Mexico for my Ph.D. in psychology. However, life often gets in the way of our plans and I had to go to work. I was fortunate enough to obtain a position as a psychologist at Temple University Hospital in Philadelphia, in the Departments of Rehabilitation Medicine and Neurology/ Neurosurgery. Temple Hospital is a very large university hospital with their own medical, dental, and pharmacy schools as well as a school for the allied health professions.

My plan was to work for one year but I remained for nearly five years. These years proved to be the happiest years of my professional life. The vast majority of the staff, including the rehabilitation physicians, the neurosurgeons, the physical and occupational therapists as well as the nurses and aides loved to teach and had a passion for learning. They were receptive to the ideas of others and aided in their implementation. They shared a united desire to offer the best treatment for the patient, even if it meant thinking out of the box. I remember when they gave me my first paycheck. I actually felt guilty thinking, *if they knew how much I loved the work, I would do it for nothing.* The patient population I worked with included paraplegics, quadriplegics, stroke patients with hemiplegia, those with spinal cord aneurysms, those with alcoholism, along with a multitude of others.

One of my earliest observations was about the patients I treated with alcoholism. When I was at Haverford State Hospital, there were 22 men and 22 women with the diagnosis of alcoholism in my unit. The majority had been abusing alcohol for most of their lives. They were all diagnosed with a psychiatric or emotional disorder. The disease concept was being advanced at that time, although excessive drinking was still considered to be a moral failing.

I was now in a medical center where some of those with alcoholism were diagnosed with an organic brain disease including a Wernicke's or Korsakoff syndrome. The syndromes were characterized by confusion, ataxia, time disorientation, and confabulation (the result of memory loss), among other symptoms. The administration of thiamin and other nutrients seemed to be standard unless the behavior warranted psychiatric intervention.

What stood out for me is that in my years at Haverford Hospital, I had never heard of the above organic brain syndromes. I believe the patients at Haverford must have received similar medical treatment, but the diagnoses in the two hospitals for the same disease were different. One emphasized the psychological and the other the medical aspects of the same illness—a form of brain damage. Remembering the 60-year-old patient who was treated for seven months with aversive conditioning, I realized that never once during this period did any of the four Ph.D. psychologists even talk about or, as far as I know, consider the man could possibly have been suffering from brain damage.

It became apparent that the diagnosis a person receives is often determined less so by the symptoms but by the environment and the social system in which they reside. The model and the beliefs, correct or incorrect, that the treating professional holds, along with communication in that particular clinical environment influences the diagnosis along with the remedial approaches.

I became determined not to be locked into entrenched approaches dominated by dogmatic opinions and beliefs, as I was responsible for those who place their trust in me. I knew I would be wrong at times, but I was determined not to be negligent. I ultimately came to understand and appreciate the biogenic, psychogenic, and sociogenic models of human behavior even more than ever before. My growing realization of the influence these three models can exert over treating professions became an impetus for writing this book.

It would be almost impossible to relate the entire range of experiences and opportunities that I had during the years I spent at Temple Hospital. There are a few that do warrant writing about, as the lessons taught are long-remembered and shaped my thinking as well as my behavior today.

As a psychologist, I was unusually lucky to make daily rounds with the head neurosurgical resident Dr. Greg Lignelli. We would see patients together at 6:45 in the morning. If he had a surgical case, I would observe his surgery. Other times, we would just visit each patient on his service and he would point out symptoms and other signs of injuries and diseases. One morning, he was examining a paraplegic patient and he demonstrated a Beevor's sign. This is a neurological sign found in paraplegics that identifies the level of injury in the spinal cord. When our rounds were over, we then rounded again with the neurosurgical residents who Dr. Lignelli taught and supervised. He then took the residents to see the same group of patients as we had just seen. We ultimately came to that paraplegic patient and Dr. Lignelli, without the hint of a smile, asked the resident physicians, "What's a Beevor's sign?" Every face in the group went blank with embarrassment. He then turned to me and asked the same question. I explained it, having just learned about it minutes before. He then said, "If a psychologist knows what that reflex is, there is no excuse for residents not knowing it." The residents never found out that this was a setup, but it never hurt me to appear intelligent. I believe his talent, in part, also resided in his undiminished passion for learning.

One of the senior neurosurgeons at Temple Hospital was Dr. Henry Wycis, who I regarded as extraordinarily gifted. He treated Parkinson's disease and the associated symptoms with stereotactic surgery, an innovation of his own design. This consisted of drilling holes in the patient's skull and inserting carefully aimed rods into the brain in order to destroy those centers that were responsible for the abnormal movement, loss of muscle control and balance characteristic of Parkinson's. These were the days before L-Dopa (Levodopa), a drug that made these surgeries unnecessary. These operations were not without risk, and it took extreme skill to perform them. I witnessed this surgery when it failed, and the results were devastating for the patient. However, at that time, I was in awe of Dr. Wycis.

Not long after I left Temple Hospital to attend the University of Pennsylvania for my Ph.D., I became familiar with the work of Dr. I. S. Cooper. He was, at that time, a young brain surgeon who had developed an alternative surgery to the stereotactic procedure called a thalamectomy. The procedure also treated movement disorders, including those of Parkinson's. The surgical risk was less and the outcomes superior to the stereotactic procedure. Despite having conclusive filmed evidence of his patients' successes, he had to endure ridicule, rejection, and vitriolic attacks. There is little doubt that he made enormous and original contributions to medicine and surgery. The prevailing thought to explain the vindictive attacks was put forth by one of his colleagues. Adrian Upton, M.D. wrote, and I quote, "A young physician can expect nothing but trouble from an important discovery made early in his career." He continued, "Such an individual would be wise to attribute his discovery to luck rather than ability." He also suggested that a pioneer should develop some physical handicap (a limp, a stutter, or an eye patch) in order to offset jealousy with sympathy. To me, this attitude reflects a march backward into the dark ages. Why should Dr. Cooper have to fight for acceptance as Galileo did in the 17th century (15)?

What was surprising for me to grasp was that Dr. Henry Wycis, a man I truly admired, was one of the attackers. In a conference, he stated that Dr. Cooper's work could not be accurate and that if "you want to learn more about Cooper's work, read it in next month's *Ladies' Home Journal*" (14). This undignified comment was unexpected and at the very least disappointing.

When I finished my Ph.D., I remember asking a psychiatrist whether I would feel differently about myself for having completed my education. He laughed and said, "Well, make up your mind whether you want to be a chief-chief or a human-chief." I'll take human-chief every time! I quickly discovered the need to question the prevailing dogmas of my own field. I, therefore, had an obligation to keep an open mind and maintain an awareness of those influences that would restrict my thinking. Everyone working in a clinical or teaching environment must struggle with resources, environmental influences, other personalities, as well as the limitations imposed by our own beliefs and experiences. Despite these pulls, we are obligated to become better at what we do.

For over 40 years, I have practiced clinical psychology and neuropsychology. I had the privilege of studying with the renowned anthropologist Dr. Ray Birdwhistell, who you will come to know better in Chapter 4. I have taught undergraduate students, graduate students, medical residents, nursing students, psychiatric residents, and even high school students. This book is, in part, written due to the encouragement I received from them.

At times, I have heard graduate students in psychology say that much of what we do is common sense. Occasionally, this may appear to be accurate, but most often nothing could be further from the truth. What passes for common sense is usually a reflection of our own beliefs that may be based upon fallacious models. Try the following on yourself. It is a question I often pose to those I teach or others who attend my lectures, but before you answer, think of the assumptions you hold.

"Who taught you to blush?"

The responses often include: "It's natural," "Nobody," "It just happens automatically," and other similar opinions. It is true, blushing is automatic. Everyone can blush throughout the world and blushing is, as we all know, a response to a social stimulus. This can be a response to an off-color joke, a response to being teased, or even to a compliment. Our parents do not sit us down and give us "blushing" lessons. How, then, do we learn this response? We are physiologically capable of blushing all over our body, but it happens that we only blush on our faces, the nape of our neck, and our hands—those areas that are seen by others. This happens through nonverbal communication that is ubiquitous and vital to every social system. This form of communication is one of the ways we acquire those models and beliefs that help us to understand our world.

Another example of a belief we may hold is our meaning of the word "dropout." For many, it suggests failure, an inability to succeed or complete something. It is as though we know what trajectory individuals should follow from the start to the finish. If they don't, they are often labeled a dropout. When we communicate this, we have denied the individual their right to level off with dignity and honor as their ability and circumstances permit.

A third example that exposes our belief system: When tall plants are crossbred with short plants of the same species, what size is the offspring of this pairing? The frequent and quick response is, "a medium-size plant." I am often amazed when I get this response, even from people who are familiar with Mendelian genetics. Most cannot relate this question to their own life experiences. For example, when a male and female mate, is the offspring something in the middle? Maybe common sense is not always enough!

Many years later, when I was on staff at Abington Memorial Hospital, a large general hospital in Abington, Pennsylvania, I saw a patient for psychological testing in the locked psychiatry unit. When I went to give the results to the referring psychiatrist, he was in his scheduled Tuesday meeting reviewing his patients with the nursing staff. Waiting for my turn to speak, I heard the psychiatrist state pejoratively, "All these patients want are sleeping pills." I spoke up and asked, why not consider using a behavioral approach to teach the patients how to sleep without medication? He said to me, "You try it" and gave me the names of two women both diagnosed with schizophrenia who shared the same room.

I was somewhat intimidated by the diagnosis, as I now had something to prove. Sitting in the room with the women, I honestly told the two of them that I needed their help. I detailed a behavior modification program that I had frequently used with patients who had severe sleeping difficulties. I asked that they honestly try the program for one week, and they both agreed to follow my suggestions. One week later, I returned to the psychiatrist's Tuesday meeting to see if the program had worked. Nursing gave their report and, of course, the night shift nurses' notes were included. It was reported the two patients had followed the program I detailed and had slept without asking for pills. As I got up to leave, I observed the psychiatrist reorder the sleeping medication for these two women. I can only assume he was wedded to the medical model and was comfortable in his belief medication was the best source of treatment. An alternative approach, even when shown to be effective, did not fit into his mindset. I can only guess at his motivation, but had to wonder how much medication is unnecessarily administered without an effort to teach patients how they might attempt to help themselves. A pill is an easier and quicker fix, and also communicates the message we are doing something. In other cases, the problem may be a lack of awareness or lack of interest as well as a lack of ability of the treating physician. I believe this physician also denied those professionals in that meeting an opportunity to learn about treatment options other than medications.

It appears the entire range of human experiences and behavior is often witnessed in hospitals. I did not fully understand nor was I willing to accept this resistance to change with its lack of receptiveness to new and potentially beneficial ideas. I was determined to tease out the dogmas in my own profession that limited effective interventions. As I mentioned in the introduction, I believe it is essential, if we are to help, that we build correctives into our own behavior by being open to multiple ways of seeing and thinking. Is this not the obligation and function of all professionals who treat or teach others? We are all dependent upon the approbations of those around us but not at the expense of truth. The following is a recent example of why questioning is a valuable asset.

Recently, I received an email from the wife of a couple that my wife and I traveled with in Europe. Her husband was exhibiting signs of dementia and she asked if I was familiar with a new device that electrically stimulated the nasal passages of individuals with dementia in order to improve cognitive functioning. The device sold for $500 and she would willingly purchase it for her husband if it might improve his memory. I reviewed the research on this mechanism and found the study consisted of five subjects who were treated with electrical nasal stimulation for a period of four weeks. Their statistics indicated positive results. The study was sponsored and performed by the company that made and sold this tool. One subject had dropped out of the study, and their supported statistics were terribly flawed. In addition, once the treatment stopped, so did any potential benefits. I emailed my impressions and the wife wisely decided against spending the $500. I felt it was important for her to question whose good was being served with this device.

Before we finish this chapter, I ask the reader to compare and contrast the attitudes and personalities reflected in the following experiences.

A 35-year-old married man with five children had been admitted to the Department of Physical Rehabilitation of Temple Hospital with cerebellar ataxia. During surgery, he had experienced oxygen deprivation, and because he had a history of alcohol use, his cerebellum was damaged. Consequently, he developed ataxia—a loss of coordination of the muscles of his extremities. If one said, "Good morning, Mr. Jones," he would turn his head and fall out of his wheelchair, as his entire body would sporadically jump. He could not eat by himself because his hand shook and trembled, making it impossible for him to get the fork or spoon to his mouth. During morning rounds, the doctors and nurses would greet him and quickly move on to the next patient. All of us were embarrassed because we had nothing to offer and we were simply helpless to treat his condition. I felt an obligation to try something for his sake as well as my own. I also felt a responsibility to his wife as she understandably expected that a hospital would help.

I believed, as I understood the function of the cerebellum, that with appropriate training I might enable the higher centers of his brain, the cerebrum, to bring some control over his ataxic condition. Three times a day, seven days a week for two weeks, Mr. Jones and I practiced relaxation with imaginal control over his ataxic movements. The training included learning to eat and walk with deliberate movements controlled by using relaxation techniques. For example, he would take his fork, put it into the food, raise it toward his mouth, pause to think and relax, and repeat the steps until the food reached his mouth. It must be pointed out that the medical staff supported my efforts, even if not convinced they would prove to be of value.

After the training, I announced Mr. Jones could walk. The entire staff of my department gathered in the large physical therapy gym as Mr. Jones was wheeled in. He then proceeded to remove his safety belt, stand, and before taking his first step he steadied himself. With the same repeated efforts at each of his steps, he managed to circumnavigate the gym. The physicians were thrilled for the patient's success, and the occasion was even filmed and videotaped. Unfortunately, Mr. Jones's insurance soon ran out and he was transferred to the massive Philadelphia General Hospital, where patients without funds were treated. I also included with his transfer a detailed description of what had been done with Mr. Jones but had little hope it would be continued. I, therefore, also included what was to be my next step had the patient remained in our hospital. This was a recommendation for two medications that I believed might be of benefit. When I suggested these medications to our physicians and I gave my justification, Dr. Lignelli again supported me stating, "Hell, we don't know any more than you do." The only report I ever received was from our social worker indicating that the physicians at Philadelphia General tried the medications with "some success."

I was lucky enough to be a teaching fellow at the University of Pennsylvania and while contemplating a topic for my dissertation, I thought about Mr. Jones. I wondered if a similar approach with modifications could be used with hyperactive children so they might develop the ability to inhibit their behavior, without medication, using self-imposed cortical control and thereby direct their attention to facilitate learning. I went to the Philadelphia school district and asked permission to conduct this study. They recommended an elementary school in West Philadelphia where teachers were known to be struggling with children they felt were not learning due to attention deficit hyperactivity disorder. Based upon my own school experience, when the teacher said "pay attention," it meant I was to fold my hands, place them on my desk, and look at her. The teacher had no idea if my mind was on the lesson or was elsewhere. When school starts, children are given a pencil and books but are really not taught how to attend or concentrate. So, I began to develop an attention training program. I felt, before implementing my ideas, it would be helpful to obtain an expert's opinion of my approach. At that time, Dr. Donald Meichenbaum was considered to be the authority and expert in modifying and training attention. One of my professors at Penn knew him and arranged for the two of us to meet. I explained my research idea in detail to him. He looked at me and stated, "it won't work" and left the room. There was no explanation as to why it would not work nor was there any encouragement to continue with my study.

I am proud to say that I did complete the initial research with success. The first-, second-, and third-graders involved in the study all demonstrated increased capacities for maintaining selective attention, and this ability continued long after the study was over. Eventually, I trained the entire student body of another Philadelphia elementary school, including students with and without special needs. The positive effects of teaching attention and concentration was equally successful with the majority of students. Dr. Meichenbaum eventually changed his focus away from training attention and has since made significant contributions to the field of cognitive behavioral therapy.

While at Penn, I took a class whose focus reflected the professor's interests—social-emotional problems that interfered with classroom learning. The students in my class were required to identify a problem that contributed to a failure to learn. I had been interested in gang violence since I was at Temple Hospital. One of my responsibilities was to tell a gang-related shooting victim, and there were many, they would never walk again. I would, after surgery, go into the recovery room and, with difficulty, give this terrible news. More often than not, there was a police officer at the patient's room because it was not unusual if a member of the gang that shot the patient found out he was alive, he or another gang member would not hesitate to come into the hospital to "finish the job." Eventually, this led to my having the first group therapy at Temple Hospital with only paralyzed gang victims. One of the patient's I was particularly fond of was an intelligent and personable young paralyzed man of 18. He eventually left the hospital in a wheelchair and as he was leaving, I apologized for not being able to do more for him. Less than a year later, I received a call from his mother letting me know that he was back in the hospital, dying, and that he wanted to see me.

He explained that he had returned to the streets and operated his gang from his wheelchair. Violence and drugs caught up with him, and these circumstances brought him to his present condition. He wanted to thank me for what I had tried to do and apologized for not listening to me earlier. We spoke for a very long time about his life. He did survive and agreed to make a video about what it was like to be part of the gang culture. However, he was afraid that gang members who worked in the hospital would object to his making a recording. Several of us carried him down a stairwell to the basement of the hospital where the video recorder had been set up. The 55-minute tape remains quite powerful as he relates life without a father and the pseudo-rewards of gang affiliations. The gang members, he believed, were male surrogates for fatherly acceptance. Indoctrination began at eight or nine years of age when they were given guns to hold for the older gang members because "the police would never search kids." He spoke about the meaninglessness of school as it bore no relationship to the lives of the inner-city students. He acknowledged his destructive behavior, use of weapons, and eventually his prison experiences. After his release, he entered the Job Corps, turned his life around, and felt he was becoming more productive. However, one Christmas while visiting his mother, he went to the store to purchase stamps and when returning home, he was stopped because he had entered another gang's turf. He tried to explain that he was no longer a gang member and was now in the Job Corp, but was still attacked. Outnumbered, he tried to fight but suddenly felt his arms drop to his sides and he fell between two cars. Awake, he looked over his shoulder and saw a former friend standing over him with a knife. He counted the five stabs that paralyzed him for life.

Needless to say, the tape was quite moving but the professor would not let me show it in class. As unbelievable as this sounds, he did not consider gang violence to be a significant part of school-related problems as it was not in the classroom. To this day, I still have no idea of what he was thinking. I told him I was going to show the tape to our class anyway, and I invited him to join us. Following the viewing of the tape, there were very few dry eyes in the room and I believe it did have an emotional impact on the professor. The tape's message is as relevant today as it was when first made. I still find it hard to believe that a college professor would have such a closed mind. But then I remembered Semmelweis.

I would be remiss if I did not include the research of Dr. Robert Kleiner, a professor of social psychology in sociology at Temple University. While studying for my master's degree, I had a research assistantship with Dr. Kleiner, who was investigating new treatment approaches for chronic backward mental patients who were residents of the Philadelphia State Hospital known as Byberry. At one time, this hospital housed 6,000 mental patients. The 36 patients in Dr. Kleiner's study had been in this hospital from 12 to 52 years, and now we were discharging them, as long as the subjects were agreeable, directly into the community. I came to the study a few days after the fall term started. The graduate students involved in the study were sociology majors except for a student in communication who videotaped the therapy sessions. I was the only psychology graduate student. During our very first meeting, Dr. Kleiner explained how the data had been collected and how we were going to proceed.

After listening, I believed there might be a more effective way to collect the data that would yield more information. Dr. Kleiner asked me to explain my ideas, and I requested additional time to think it through. The next day, I outlined my thinking about our observation and recording of patient interactions. Dr. Kleiner agreed that my suggestion for collecting data would provide more information than previously obtained and that he was willing to start the research anew. I was not directly involved with the group therapies that were conducted by hospital-affiliated psychologists. My responsibility along with the other graduate assistants was to record observations through a two-way mirror.

The hospital no longer exists as many free-standing mental hospitals in Pennsylvania have long been closed and torn down. When these hospitals were open, the process of discharge involved releasing the patients directly into the community as soon as they demonstrated some improvement in their symptoms. This traditional discharge approach was proven to be a failure as statistics indicted the recidivism rate was almost at 100 percent. The halfway house discharge was the next approach. Patients who were considered well enough to leave the hospital but not independently enter society would reside for a period of time in a halfway program designed to introduce them slowly back into the community. This approach had a 30 percent success rate.

Based upon these dismal statistics, Dr. Kleiner obtained a two-year federal grant to investigate different approaches. He viewed things differently from the prevailing time-honored models of treatment and discharge. Therapy had not been effective in this population, and he conceived of a new research paradigm he called the enabler model. He wanted individuals from the Philadelphia area to work with and even live with patients who would now be returning directly into community living. He advertised for individuals with a high school education to be part of the investigation. The patients were discharged from the hospital into apartments and divided up into four treatment groups. If a patient or subject was overwhelmed by the loss of the security of the hospital, he or she was free to return. Very few did. The groups were divided as follows with three residents in each apartment:

Group 1—The enablers resided in the same apartment with the subjects and the subjects received group therapy.

Group 2—The enablers lived with the subjects but only the enablers received group therapy.

Group 3—The subjects lived alone in their apartment and were visited by their enablers. The subjects received the group therapy.

Group 4—The subjects lived alone in their apartment and were visited by their enablers. The enablers in these groups received the therapy.

Therapy, in all groups, focused on the understanding of the manifestations of mental illness along with self-help strategies. A remarkable 70 percent success rate was achieved in Group 2.

In this group, the enablers lived with the subjects and received the group therapy. The results were impressive that the federal government funded the study for an additional five years.

I was with Dr. Kleiner for two memorable years and learned to respect and admire his integrity, honesty, intelligence, and openness to other's ideas. It is to his credit the outcome of his study became the treatment model for chronically ill patients in the country of Norway. Dr. Kleiner was exceptional in that he, the teacher, and he, the pupil, were within the same man—an individual who thought about and embraced change if it benefited others.

I love teaching and learning but feel obligated to say that after 10 years of college, the majority of my courses and teachers did not have the impact on me that I would have liked. There were, however, a few professors who I will always be deeply indebted to as they had a tremendous influence on my thinking and consequently the course of my life. I can never thank them enough. When I taught graduate students, I would suggest before signing up for their next semester's courses, they consider interviewing their prospective professors for the next semester to get an impression of whether the professor and the course would meet their expectations. I added, if you went to McDonald's and a rotten hamburger was served to you, what would you do? I stressed that what these students would do for a two-dollar hamburger, they should also do for their education. If the professor did not take the time to respond to their questions, I advised them to take another course unless there was no other option.

If you are lucky to be in a stimulating environment, take the opportunity to knock on as many doors as possible and let them know about your passion to learn. Your goal is not to master their field, but to increase your ability to understand what they do and expand your horizons through new ideas, concepts, and approaches.

These suggestions are not presented in a cavalier or Pollyannaish manner but rather to support the reader in their efforts to become informed and bring a science-based investigation to new knowledge. This will facilitate an openness to build correctives into outdated and ineffective models of human behavior. Learning is terribly exciting if it impacts your thinking and your ability to reason. You may find that nature is simpler than our thoughts about nature, but the difficult part is to understand this simplicity. I believe Dr. Richard Feynman shared this view. So, if you do, you are in very good company.

Einstein stressed that science is one of the most precious things we have not because it guarantees absolute truths but, rather, it is a self-correcting method to advance our understanding of the social and natural world. If we are to self-correct, we must also overcome the limitations fixed by our own beliefs. This is our next step in our journey together.

CHAPTER 2

The Biogenic Model

The reader will note the three models to be presented in this and subsequent chapters are interrelated and interdependent. The medical, or biogenic, model is the one held in highest esteem by our society. At the foundation of the biogenic model is the belief that symptoms of illness have their origins in physical causes. If the cause is not readily apparent to the treating physician, then various diagnostic tests may be ordered. The goal of the biogenic model is to determine the problem and avenues for addressing it with medication, surgery, a change in lifestyle, or some other type of intervention. In most cases this may be enough, but as one ages this approach becomes more complicated.

While medicine is a science, the practice of medicine is an art; sciences do not generate arts directly out of themselves. It takes an open, inventive, and moral individual to become this kind of artist. The focus in this chapter is to suggest that physicians often lack an appreciation or an understanding of the psychogenic and sociogenic models that also aid in the understanding of illness. This omission can weaken the efficacy of treatment outcomes. It bears repeating that medicine is but one model in the understanding and treatment of human disease and suffering. Its efficacy could be enhanced if practitioners were aware of and receptive to the other complementary models. It is essential to remember that the question we ask determines the answer we receive. If we only ask a medical question, we will only get a medical answer

There is little doubt that most practicing physicians are intelligent and talented. I am in awe of some of the medical miracles I have witnessed. However, for most practitioners, medicine has changed. Presently, there are tremendous pressures imposed upon physicians stemming from hospital-dominated and -owned practices to newer Medicare and managed health care guidelines. Medicine has become a numbers game. Today, one hears a common complaint, "My doctor spends almost no time with me." Given these alterations in practice, it is essential that physicians become aware of the full impact on patients. I cannot overstate the importance of the relationship between the physician and the patient in determining physical and emotional outcomes. This chapter is devoted to illuminating the importance of this communication.

I remember, as a child, our physician made house calls. He would sit on my bed and assure me that I would mend. His behavior engendered a most comforting feeling, and while the illness may have been self-limiting, this reassurance was every bit as important as the medication he prescribed.

I also recall Dr. Joseph Bitman, the pediatrician for both of our sons. His first visit, after their birth and discharge from the hospital, was in our apartment. He initiated these visits. It not only impressed me and my wife, but also his behavior engendered a sense of trust and caring. After his examination, we had coffee and he explained that every first visit with his newborn patients was at their homes because he felt it was vital to get an impression of the environment in which the infant was being raised. His greatest frustration was that his large practice often prevented him from communicating the worth of this approach to his colleagues.

Most of us have heard of a behavior known as the hands-on phenomenon. Suppose a physician comes to your hospital room and says, "Your labs are great, the surgery was a success, your medication is perfect, and you are mending." The patient will likely be thrilled and mend in time. However, if the physician says exactly the same thing but holds your hand while using the identical words, that patient will experience an increase in leucocytes (white blood cells), which are responsible for fighting infection. This touched patient will, in all probability, mend quicker.

The communication of caring is tremendously enhanced through touch. When was the last time a physician touched you? Now, teachers and other professionals are quite cautious before they even consider touching another person's hand or shoulder. Perhaps we should not have thrown out the values of the past but reinterpreted them in the light of the present.

I wanted to understand how this phenomenon worked. When an infant is fed by his or her mother, whether by breast or bottle, leucocytes are necessary to digest the milk. The relationship between touch and the generating of leucocytes, established through Pavlovian learning, explained the hands-on miracle that continues for the rest of the human lifespan. I was, later to learn, that I was only partially correct and there were additional nonverbal mechanisms indelibly established in our earliest days (12).

It appears to begin in infancy or possibly even in utero. The tactile stimuli from suckling produces neural signals that travel to the upper brain via the spinothalamic tract. They reach the upper and immediate brain: first the sensory cortices, then the limbic system, the prefrontal cortex, and finally the hypothalamus. In the hypothalamus, the descending neural signals are responsible for the release of oxytocin into the bloodstream. The time required for this to happen is 15 seconds. When a mother sees or hears the baby cry, oxytocin can also trigger the release of milk beyond the mother's conscious control. The effects of oxytocin determine our interactions, especially social interactions, for the remainder of our lives. The primary way of obtaining oxytocin is through positive relationships. Dr. Tallie Baram, a child neuroscientist, found that a mother's caress can trigger the release of oxytocin, and this improves cognition and resilience to stress in a baby's developing brain. The mother's touch literally prevents the release of stress hormones that are neurotoxic. Recognizing this, orphan infants in England and Ireland that otherwise would not have been touched are permitted during the day to be held and coddled by female prisoners. Both groups have derived significant benefits from this arrangement (34).

Until the discovery of quinine, the placebo was the one of the most important medicines we had. Simply defined, a placebo is a medicine without an active ingredient. The use of placebos was widely considered effective for centuries (33). By the 19th century, it was common practice to use placebos when other medical treatments had been exhausted; they were also used for patients who were simply anxious about their health. It is true that many doctors felt they were deceiving their patients. There was the concern that if the patients found out there was no active substance in the medication, the doctor would run the risk of being thought of as a quack. However, most physicians at the time felt placebos were still too useful to give up.

The father of the modern placebo movement is Henry Beecher, who defined the use of the placebo as a medical treatment. He became interested in the placebo effect as an army physician during the battles of WWII. Injured soldiers were injected with a salt solution, because morphine was in short supply and unavailable. The soldiers reported a decrease in pain and generally felt better after an injection with the placebo. The positive effect of the placebo was enhanced if administered by an empathetic and attentive medic. As long as the patient had confidence in their care provider and believed they were getting the best treatment available, their recovery was enhanced. It was patently obvious that a person's mental state played a central role in the placebo effect.

In 1955, Dr. Beecher wrote a paper titled, "The Powerful Placebo." He surmised that in certain instances placebos produced "gross physical change(s) that could exceed those attributable to potent pharmacological action." Thirty to 40 years later, some physicians in American medicine began to wonder if the sugar pills used in the randomized controlled trial studies might be more biologically and therapeutically significant than was initially apparent. Thirty percent of all patients, whether they are in a hospital or in their home, are placebo reactors. If the physician or nurse administering the placebo believes it is the real medication, the number of placebo reactors increases to between 60 and 70 percent. This means the act of giving out the pill is every bit as important as the pill itself. The placebo reaction remains part of all therapeutics in use (28).

We know that pain creates, among other things, neurotoxins. It is estimated that 85 percent of the elderly experience some kind of pain. In order to control pain, physicians have turned to opioids.

In the late 1990s, pharmaceutical companies reassured the medical establishment that patients would not become addicted to opioid pain relievers. Unfortunately, increased prescriptions led to wide-scale use and abuse of prescription opioids. Now, we are in a national crisis with overdoses accounting for more than 42,000 opioid deaths in 2016 alone. More than three out of five drug overdoses involve an opioid, and these deaths are continuing to increase in the US (51). During this same year, opioid abuse had removed more than one million individuals from the work force at an estimated cost of $95 billion (39). CNN recently reported there have been 67,000 deaths as the result of opioid overdoses. New, synthetic opioids are even more potent than heroin and other prescription pain medications. During my 40 years working in hospitals and other medical settings, I have, when appropriate, advocated using placebos for pain. This suggestion has been rejected in the vast majority of facilities, because it was considered illegal to trick or fool patients. I refuse to accept this excuse and, given the historical use of placebos, believe they are, in many cases, a viable alternative to opioids. Might we not, in light of the opioid deaths, rethink our objections to what I believe is a legitimate medical approach?

In one medical center, I suggested the use of a placebo to the treating physician because the patient was taking very high doses of opioids for pain control. The pharmacy made a capsule of an inert substance that was placed into a blister pack with the name "Cebo" on the container. I instructed the patient to take three of these new pills for pain every six hours and left the medication in her room. I added, if three powerful capsules did not control her pain, she was free to take a fourth capsule. I had observed that when hospital patients are in control of their own pain medication, they tend to be more conservative. Within the first day of using Cebos, the patient had total remission of her pain. One day, I received a phone call from the attending physician who said that a nurse told the patient what was in the capsule. He pleaded with me to tell the patient that I was to blame for tricking her. I confessed to the patient and explained my reasons for suggesting its use. The woman thanked me, and together we laughed about the Cebos. I have had several additional successes like this one.

On another occasion, I wanted to try a more Pavlovian approach to the same problem of intense pain. This time, I had the pharmacy, with the physician's support, make up a solution of water, cherry syrup, and mint flavor. Because depression is often associated with pain, an antidepressant and narcotic for pain were added to the solution. This time, I told the patient exactly what I was going to do. I told him that he would continue to drink the cocktail, but I was going to decrease and eventually eliminate the narcotic and the antidepressant. The cocktail was to retain its red color, taste, and smell. After three weeks, the cocktail had no more narcotic or antidepressant, and the pain was controlled. I believe the association of color, smell, and taste elicited his own endorphins—chemicals that inhibit the communication of pain signals. While not claiming this approach is the solution to replace analgesics or is a panacea to eliminate pain, I am asking for an open investigation to the possibility of using the mechanisms of the human body to help limit the abuse of addictive drugs.

It is equally important to educate the patient as well as the physician about alternative methods of treatment. Patient expectations need to be shifted so they no longer believe that a pill is the only solution. An indication of one shift in thinking is the use of medical marijuana for pain management and pain control. Recent research suggests that it has been beneficial in replacing opioids for pain control without the untoward effects (24).

Another sign of a shift in thinking is that some are looking at pain as part of a communication system. If a patient with intractable pain is given a PET scan, the pain centers in the brain can be visualized. It has been shown if a patient in pain and a patient who is pain-free share a hospital room, both of their pain centers will be illuminated by a PET scan. The pain-free individual does not feel the pain, but there is an emotional connection with the one in pain. There does seem to be a communication of pain, which will be expanded upon in Chapter 4 when we discuss SYNC and other forms on nonverbal communication. I believe it is essential to remember that each cell in our body is related to our entire social system. This is a relatively new finding and will take time in order to understand its influences on and consequences for our interventions.

Given the above examples, I am asking physicians and others, regardless of their field, to overcome the limitations imposed by their own specialties. It is important to remember that knowledge in our society is held by individuals from many disciplines. This is an increasing necessity as there has been an exponential growth of scientific material and knowledge. In the 1700s, there were fewer than 10 scientific journals. By 1800 there were about 100, in 1850 there were 1,000, and by 1900 there were 10,000. Today, there are in excess of 100,000 with global scientific output and computing capabilities (36). We live in a jungle of knowledge, and not everything in the jungle is worthwhile or genuine. No scientist can be familiar with the vastness of this material. One of the consequences in medicine has been an unprecedented increase in disciplinary specialization. It is a truism that physicians as well as others in the helping fields would benefit from working with other disciplines in a timely manner and not just when they perceive they have nothing left to offer.

I was working in a physical rehabilitation hospital and was asked to see a young woman of 21 years of age who had her right leg and hip removed because of an osteosarcoma (bone cancer). Due to her age, the surgeon had given her the option of this radical surgery or a less invasive procedure where the tumor would be removed and the leg radiated. He was puzzled by her insistence on the surgery that removed the leg and hip, and I was asked to shed some light on why she made the decision she had. I responded, "Why didn't you ask me to speak with her before the surgery?" After spending some time with the patient, she reached under her hospital pillow and pulled out some magazines that suggested men were more sexually attracted to disabled women.

This was her reason for electing the radical, life-altering surgery that might have been prevented had I seen the patient prior to the operation. A simple shift in thinking and timing may have dramatically changed the outcome, but an openness to change is not always easy. Society can only benefit if we strive to build correctives into our thinking and actions.

I had been Chief of Psychology for 25 years in another rehabilitation department when a new, inexperienced medical director was appointed. One morning while making rounds, I suggested she use a stimulant medication for a particular stroke patient. I understand and respect the fact that the physician is ultimately responsible for the consequences of administering all medications. However, without asking about my background or my reasons for suggesting that particular medication, she immediately responded, "We never do that." I proposed that we consult with another specialist in the field of stroke rehabilitation about the merit of my suggestion. She selected and phoned a well-known physician from a major rehabilitation center in Philadelphia. He completely agreed with my recommendation and indicated that the medication is frequently used given the symptoms our patient exhibited. After the call, the medicine was administered and the patient eventually improved. However, the medical director was apparently upset and ordered the nurses to take rectal temperatures every morning on all 24 patients in our unit. Needless to say, this time she had to deal with the blow back from the nursing staff, and I was sure this time she had no expert to phone.

I witnessed a young physician walk into the room of a newly paralyzed patient and say, "You will never walk again," and then immediately exit the room leaving that individual in an emotional crisis. This physician either lacked the sensitivity or training, or was so terribly uncomfortable with the task he had to perform, he communicated a devastating message to an unprepared patient. I believe he had not been taught that patients frequently do not ask questions they are fearful of having answered. During the years I worked with spinal cord injuries, it was extremely rare, if ever, a patient asked me directly about their chances of walking again. They would ask questions all around this issue but seldom this specific question. I learned to wait until they were ready for the answer, and they invariably guided my behavior. It is also ironic that in our society, the onus of teaching others how to be comfortable with a disability falls upon the person with the disability. We simply have not been taught how to feel at ease with many types of handicaps. Our discomfort is then communicated to those who are in some way different. An openness to other disciplines would have provided this physician with knowledge that could have guided his interactions with patients.

My father had terminal cancer that started in his stomach and had spread to his throat. He was unable to swallow water but, despite this, he remained alert. Several days before he passed, I was in the hospital shaving him. Right outside of his room were two physicians debating should they or should they not tell my father he was dying. My father was not deaf, nor was the other terminal patient who shared his room. I went out to the physicians and asked them to leave, explaining that it was my responsibility to communicate to my dad the end was very near. I waited until my father asked me what I felt his future was. I said," What do you think?" His response was, "The grim reaper." I nodded and replied yes. When I asked if he was frightened, he replied, "The Bible promises three score and ten." My dad was 74 years old. I relate this with the hope that those of you who read this book will challenge the experts should you feel their opinion or behavior is questionable. If you feel strongly about your belief, do not be afraid to stand up to authorities or experts and express your own thoughts. In my father's case, one had to wonder if those doctors considered the impact of their deliberation on the patient. A richer understanding of the human condition depends on the courage of those who dare to leave themselves open to think and act differently.

Compare the above with another experience that I had with Dr. Lignelli in the intensive care unit on the neurosurgical floor. On one occasion, he said, "I need your help placing some catheters into the brain of a patient." The patient had been operated on that day but remained comatose. The injury had caused some of the frontal bones of his skull to penetrate his brain. I was terrified and stated, "Remember, I'm a psychologist and we don't do this." He indicated I was the only one in the unit. This left me little choice. I swabbed the patient's head with an antiseptic as Dr. Lignelli took out a sterile hand drill making several surgical holes in the patient's cranium. I positioned and held the patient's head while the catheters were inserted with the purpose of releasing the infection in his brain. Thin fluid eventually squirted out through the inserted tubes. We then attempted several spinal taps, but the infected spinal fluid was too thick, so nothing was released by the catheters. Dr. Lignelli looked into the patient's eyes and with sadness accurately predicted the time of his passing. This experience influenced me in several ways.

I became aware that when one is caught up in and participates in the event, one ceases to be afraid. My initial terror disappeared when I became part of the experience. It helped explain an observation that the worst of times often brings out the best in others. When Dr. Lignelli looked at the patient and sadly stated, "What have I saved," I had the overwhelming feeling that he was honoring the patient by recognizing his place in the community of men. Dr. Lignelli was one of those men who had taken on the responsibility of sharing his gifts with others. There was never any doubt in my mind that he felt uncomfortable at the sight of unmerited misery. This is why he returned to try to help this patient. I know he took pride in believing each individual had something to offer. I began to understand why after rounds, we would hold a kind of communion and talk of life and not death.

When I was still at Temple University Hospital, I was asked to evaluate a patient with intractable pain. The neurology workup could not reveal any particular organic cause. I was then asked if I had something to contribute to their understanding of the problem. The patient happened to have been my professor of cognitive psychology at Temple University as well as my past advisor. She was frequently absent from her lectures. The class, instead of leaving the room, would ask me to lecture about the subject, as I had a fair understanding of the material even though I was also one of the students. This may have bred some resentment in the professor; when she returned, she was not always pleasant to me. Now, in the hospital, I was obligated to see her. The roles had been reversed. I went to her hospital room but could not bring myself to knock on the door. I thought she was still the professor, and I could not stand at the foot of her bed and look down upon her without diminishing her or myself. I approached the referring physician and explained why I was unable to answer this consult and he completely understood. Several weeks later, she passed away from an undetected cancer. To this day, I remain eternally grateful that I did not knock on that door. I ask those who practice the medical model to remember it is just that, a model. It should be implemented not only with intelligence but also flexibility and sensitivity.

Dr. Birdwhistell pointed out when the State of Israel was 25 years old, the doctors went on strike. For all practical purpose, except for dire emergencies, there was little medical treatment. During the 30 days of the strike, there were no deaths and illness dropped to an all-time low in Tel Aviv. When the strike ended, deaths returned to a pre-strike level, as did illness. These facts should prompt us to consider the communication of life and death. One possible explanation is that we know our brain oscillates and can synchronize with the brains of others to influence our behavior (47). This will be expanded upon in Chapter 4.

Anthropologists have made some interesting observations about family patterns of illness. Often a mother will not permit herself to become ill until the last child is married. At times, it is not uncommon to see one family member elected to be sick for the entire family. These observations are not written in stone but reflect patterns of illness observed in our culture (6).

When my brother was married, his wife's grandmother could not attend the ceremony as she was in the hospital. As the result of her age and a severely damaged left ventricle of her heart, she should have died. However, this woman clung to life until she knew her granddaughter was married. As soon as the ceremony was over, my brother and his bride went to the hospital to show the grandmother the marriage had taken place. Less than an hour later, she passed away. Others have told me similar stories. We need to strive to understand the communication of life, death, and illness. It affects all of us in varied ways at different times.

Some years ago, I gave a lecture to a small group of assistant prison wardens. I told them that solitary confinement, used to reduce aggressive behavior, often produced hypoglycemia. This condition is often associated with increases in aggression. They indicated they had never been made aware of this possibility. The *AARP Bulletin*, August 2018, reported that eight million adults age 50 and older are affected by isolation. Prolonged isolation is indicated to be a significant risk factor for poor health—an impact equivalent to smoking 15 cigarettes a day.

I feel it is reasonable to assume that while one might live in a populated neighborhood, an individual might still feel emotionally disconnected from friends, family, and the community. Might this perceived sense of isolation be, in part, responsible for some of our social problems? I believe this is the case particularly with belligerent behaviors. Medicine is obligated to consider the role of environmental interactions as they influence biologic changes within individuals. The high incidence of diabetic-related issues within the inner-city populations may be another example of environmental influence on one's biology. This cannot all be explained by diet or the lack of exercise alone. Many studies, including a large one at Johns Hopkins, have demonstrated that unhappiness in children can stunt growth.

In 1825, Sir Astley Cooper wrote, and I quote, "Anxiety, bereavement, or frustration could help to create the physical climate which left the body prey to cancer" (27). The Pasteur notion that microbes invade the body and cause illness can no longer be taken as the only explanatory model. I have witnessed many mothers care for their sons dying of AIDS. They were unaffected even without the use of suggested medical precautions.

I believe medicine has a major role to play in the understanding and remediation of social problems. To accomplish this, I encourage all medical professionals to demonstrate a willingness to keep an open mind about what transpires between two people as they function in their social systems.

How often was the science of disease behavior discussed in seminars? I have taught classes for family practice residents who acknowledged that they were unfamiliar with this science. For example, at times, when a bacterium or virus invades the body, the first response is a complex series of events. IL-1 cells, produced by macrophages, cause a slight fever but also can bring alterations in behavior. An individual can become irritable, nasty, and withdrawn. When this happens in a hospital, nursing home, or a personal care facility, a psychiatrist is often consulted. The change in behavior can serve an adaptive function within the social system. It isolates us from others. In Africa, this apparent evolutionary adaptation has been used to explain how particular tribes infected with the AIDS virus have isolated themselves due to their illness. This aggression serves to keep other tribes away from them, thereby protecting neighboring tribes from the spread of the disease. When I'm consulted about a change in behavior, I first make an attempt to rule out a medical or an adaptive issue before assuming it is a functional problem.

Evolutionary biology is a new science that also adds to our understanding of the human condition. An example of this science addresses low hemoglobin—the protein that transports oxygen to the tissues. Under most circumstances, low hemoglobin would be a cause of concern during a physical examination. However, in some third world countries, where the population is exposed to diseases, low hemoglobin is not unusual as blood iron is sequestered in the liver to deny the invading bacteria this vital element. During one lecture, a medical resident from the

Philippines said every time she has to take a physical examination in the US, she has to convince the examining physician her low hemoglobin is "normal for her." Another more commonly recognized example is the occasional utility of a fever (6).

Morning sickness has long been considered an unfortunate side effect of pregnancy. The nausea, however, coincides with the period of rapid tissue differentiation when fetal development is most vulnerable to interference by toxins. Margie Profet theorized that the nausea of pregnancy is an adaptation whereby the mother protects the fetus from exposure to toxins from strong-tasting and possible harmful substances. Her results revealed that women with more nausea were less likely to suffer miscarriages. Of course, additional studies are needed to evaluate her findings (53). Again, holding alternative models enables us to expand our capacity to ask different questions.

According to the Centers for Disease Control, the number of hospital patients in the US who acquire a staphylococcus infection with an accompanying unacceptable mortality rate is about two million. The hospitals' infection control teams are quite diligent in their attempts to curtail these outbreaks, as are most of the hospital staff. The washing of hands is of prime importance in halting this disease. The problem is not the lack of knowledge but rather one of compliance. It is of paramount importance that physicians monitor other physicians, nurses observe other nurses, and patients ask those who enter their room, "have you washed your hands?" A short time ago, a number of physicians traded their ties for bow ties. This was an attempt to control the spread of infection. It was considered that ties may touch bed covers, inadvertently passing germs from patient to patient. It now appears that it is easier to forego ties altogether. We all bear in the responsibility of stopping this unnecessary infection. Almost sounds like Semmelweis again, i.e. compliance! Speaking of compliance, the *British Journal of Nutrition* found that starting each day with a glass of water improves one's mood and reduces depression.

Ongoing efforts to expand the capabilities of all staff in medical facilities is essential. This can only enhance the treatment of and understanding of those with whom they work. "Staff infections" (staff, not staph) might be reduced. By this, I mean it may help to control the frustration that staff often face when dealing with noncompliant patients or the frustration that derives from the recognition, "I couldn't do anything to save that person."

I also believe that professional staff might improve the well-being of their patients by recognizing the impact of external hospital factors. Melatonin is often prescribed in nursing homes, hospitals, rehabilitation centers, and the like as an aid for sleep. However, blue light degrades the effect of this hormone and renders it useless. Blue light emanates from our cell phones, televisions, and other electronic devices. Red night lights can improve vision and therefore might reduce falls, especially in the elderly. Blue, green, or full spectrum bulbs in a patient's room would help them remain awake. Safety, alertness, and increased endurance are common goals of physical therapy. The use of lighting to enhance these goals will likely be ignored if it is not a part of the therapist's training.

It is important to encourage patients to ask their physician about additional treatments for their condition. For example, transcranial magnetic stimulation, a relatively benign procedure is approved by Medicare to treat Parkinson's disease. If the hospital you are in does not offer this procedure or your physician prefers other treatments, you are not likely to hear about it. The same procedure now has a relatively long history of treating depression. We know that 25 percent of depressed patients may never respond to traditional antidepressants. For 30 years, I have been on the staff of a rather large hospital in the psychiatric inpatient department. To my knowledge, the use of transcranial magnetic stimulation to treat depression has never been suggested despite its reported success rate in other hospitals. While the procedure may be expensive and may not be presently covered by all insurances for depression, the patient should be able to choose a treatment that might prove beneficial (27).

The surgeon Dr. Atul Gawande writes in his book *Better: A Surgeon's Notes on Performance* that "ordinary pneumonia remains the fourth most common cause of death in affluent countries." This, in part, is because pneumonias have become more virulent and also because medical personnel often delay timely treatment. He points out that if the correct antibiotic is started within four hours of arrival to the hospital, patients are less likely to die.

However, the time that elapses between the patient's decision to go to the hospital and the administering of medication often exceeds the four-hour time window. I do not feel it is unreasonable, given what is at stake, that doctors and nurses look at their results and then alter their behavior to achieve better outcomes. One way of facilitating this is for emergency rooms to compare their incidences of successes and failures with those of their peers in other facilities. This will shed light on the hospital's perception of whether they are as good as they believe they are (21). These issues exemplify a major theme of this book, namely building correctives into beliefs. To become better at what you do is a perpetual but worthwhile endeavor.

Modern science has turned the experience of aging and dying into a process managed by the medical community. Good doctors make every attempt to treat the illness but are often unaware that isolation is a sequela of illness. It is important to develop an awareness that when a patient is truly ill, they have no assurances of anything and may truly feel alone. We have seen that isolation can have a significant biological impact on an individual. I have witnessed the effect of isolation on individuals in communities, in hospitals, and in long-term facilities. The experience of advanced aging and death now largely takes place in hospitals and nursing homes. This means we have allowed our final days to be controlled by the orders of medicine, technology, and strangers (20). The issues surrounding the experience of aging and mortality are the subject of this book's final chapter.

Medicine often confuses treatment with care. Its concern when working with the aged is the repair of health more than nourishment of the soul. Specific goals such as those associated with activities of daily living often take priority over the emotional impact of age and illness. It is essential to be aware that every significant crisis also impacts family members in various ways. They are often left to seek out answers to questions about their loved one. When they do, it is usually with measured steps, as though they are afraid to impose upon the physician or social worker. Repeated family meetings with updates has proven to be of benefit to the concerned individuals as well the reputation of the facility itself. The impact on the family must be recognized in order to establish the communication of caring. At times, silence can be deafening to children as well as adults.

I would take my mother to have her chemotherapy for lung cancer at a well-respected cancer center. We waited together until she was taken for her infusions. To keep my mind occupied, I would write notes on what I was observing. The following words mirror my attempt to deal with her illness and its impact on me:

> Nasal tubes, white gauzes, lip patches seemed incongruous with the gold balls held by a red ribbon and a cardboard wreath wishing you a Merry Christmas. As you open the door to the examination rooms, not even a brightly lit and decorated Christmas tree, in the center of a large lobby, is noticed as you look from face to

> face trying to read each story. No matter how many people are waiting, the noise never seems to increase. An almost silence is only disturbed by a nurse calling a name. This is the signal to disappear behind the door with a cardboard wreath.

My mother had an esteemed oncologist as her physician. He was a pleasant person who clearly had a sincere interest in his patients. However, he never once asked, "How are you, and how is your family doing?" When people are not asked to share their thoughts or concerns, they have no recourse but to reflect on their own. This may be a most important moment when a professional could offer support. I believe my mother's physician had some concerns about her family, but the words were never spoken. I did not need them, but I could not help but think of those families that did. We live in a social system, a community, and family members share the fear, pain, and uncertainty of their loved ones.

When I did attention training with second graders, I would often take the opportunity to talk with them informally. I asked one of the boys what he wanted to be when he grew up. Like any seven-year-old boy, he replied, "a fireman or policeman." He then continued, "but I won't make it." I had no idea what he meant and so I asked, "Why?" He replied, "I'll probably be shot." This seven-year-old had little hope for any future. When I talk about the communication of caring, I cannot help but think of my little friend Kevin and all of those other children who permitted me to share time with them for a brief but meaningful period of my life. I can only hope that changes in our medical model have something to offer other seven-year-old youngsters and the social system that shapes them.

Another problem that should be acknowledged and addressed by physicians is the issue of sex. More than just the urologist, it is the responsibility of all medical professionals working in senior care facilities to deal with this behavior. Sexuality, intimacy, and aging are legitimate medical concerns. Pro-erections drugs (Viagra, Cialis) are a valuable resource. Intimacy can continue to be satisfying when the man and woman share a pleasure-oriented sexual style and not necessarily a performance-oriented approach. Sexuality involves the communication of affection through a sensual, playful, erotic touch, and not obligatory intercourse. Sex is about the sharing of pleasure. Aging brings about expected physical changes along with possible illnesses. Both men and women may have issues with body image, physical discomfort, and acceptance of the many changes associated with growing older. These are just some of the issues physicians should thoughtfully address to help individuals realize that aging is not necessarily a loss but a change in sexuality. Healthy and respectful sexual relationships can significantly aid in the reduction of isolation and help support improvements in physical well-being. Medical advice, especially when delivered by a physician, can reduce discomfort in women and contextualize changes in sexual performance for men (50).

Widowed men and women often seek partners with whom they can share trips, meals, and social events. However, when it comes to intimacy, guilt over past marriages, the opinions of their children, and personal insecurities often become issues. Here, the physician may feel comfortable consulting a sexual counselor, social worker, or psychologist to be part of the treatment team. In almost every senior facility where I have worked, I have dealt with heterosexual as well as homosexual relationships with honesty and respect for the needs of the involved couples. With that said, I have always believed that physicians should play an increased role in dealing with relationship issues.

In the late 1960s, cardiologists began to notice that stress played an important role in heart disease. Daily stress and tensions associated with functioning in our complex society have been observed to cause dangerously elevated blood pressure in a significant percentage of the population. Dr. Herbert Benson, a Harvard cardiologist, eventually developed the concept of the relaxation response to treat hypertension. Because relaxation was associated with transcendental meditation, many of his Harvard colleagues thought he was injuring his professional status. Eventually, he wrote *The Relaxation Response* (2). This book gives the justification for and step-by-step instructions to help guide the reader in reducing hypertension and other stress-related problems. Despite the tendency of medicine at times to be intolerant, *The Relaxation Response* has sold in excess of five million copies (28). Dr. Benson's approach must be considered a legitimate medical technique.

Shortly after I graduated from the University of Pennsylvania, I held a position at the Presbyterian hospital that is now part of Penn's medical network. As a way to supplement income, I rented a small office for my psychology practice. One patient referred to me was a professional football player. He had failed his pre-season physical and was not permitted to play because of severe essential hypertension. Although he was being treated with medication, he sought counseling with me because he was terrified his career was over and that his medical condition portended something worse. After several sessions, I decided to teach him to reduce his own high blood pressure through relaxation and biofeedback. I phoned his physician and asked that we might work together to achieve this end. The physician rejected my suggestion leaving us to work on our own.

I began teaching him imaginal focused relaxation; my hope was that it would facilitate a more rapid response. I also utilized a small biofeedback appliance that would convert the tiny electrical signals (microvolts) given off by the body into audible sounds. The training involved teaching him to reach deep states of relaxation that correlated with reductions in blood pressure. If he was not sufficiently relaxed, a sound would be heard stemming from the electrical output due to muscle tension. When he obtained a deeper state of relaxation, the sound would stop. Each session involved teaching him to achieve deeper and deeper relaxation. Blood pressure readings were documented in order to measure progress. There was a clear correlation between his ability to relax and the consistent lowering of his blood pressure.

After several months of training, my patient reported that his physician was reducing his medication. Although that football season was lost, my patient returned to playing professional football the following year without the need for medication. It did take the better part of a year to accomplish this goal. I found in this case as well as others that the relaxation response maintained itself once acquired.

There is little doubt that stress impacts one's health. It is responsible for increases in the number of heart attacks, type 2 diabetes, gastrointestinal problems, and depression. Chronic stress impairs the body's ability to fight inflammation, which is a precursor to many illnesses. This leaves us more susceptible to infections and is possibly linked to forms of dementia. The mind-body connection is quite potent and while it might not be able to repair a damaged heart, it can help fortify an immune system. Relaxation training might be used as an alternative to medication or in tandem with it to reduce stress and associated symptoms.

The importance of music therapy in stroke rehabilitation is woefully neglected. If you have ever worked with an aphasic patient who is unable to speak, try having them sing. Dr. Oliver Sacks in his book *Musicophilia* stresses the critical role music plays in our brain's health. Many times, I have asked an expressive aphasic patient to sing "Happy Birthday" with me. When they hear themselves sing, it is accompanied by an expression of renewed hope. The alliance of music therapy and medicine in the treatment of stroke patients is of paramount importance.

An obvious hurdle is payment for music therapy. This would require that the medical community educate the insurance carriers about the benefits of this therapy and other alternative treatment techniques for the purpose of enhancing patient outcomes. Reduction in recovery times would be of obvious benefit to both the patient and the insurance carrier (42).

There is little doubt that the practice of medicine is going through a rapid period of change. Presently, a typical clinical visit lasts just 15 minutes. A nurse or nurse's aide checks your vitals, and you wait until the physician comes in and opens up his or her laptop. Medications are reviewed, complaints noted, tests are ordered, and electronic prescriptions are sent. In the near future, advancing technology will enable the patient to be able to monitor their own vitals through a temporary tattoo (epidermal electronics) that captures biometric data, the goal being the physician will be able to spend more time with the patient. However, the present reality is hospital administrations are more concerned with the number of patients seen rather than the quality of treatment.

Virtual care, also known as telehealth, involves the remote diagnosis and treatment of patients by medical experts who are miles or even continents away. While saving money, it does provide quality of care for patients who might not otherwise have access to specialists. For older Americans, it has the potential of putting a virtual doctor right into the homes of patients. Coupled with this are impressive advances in medical treatment. They include medical 3D printing of human organs and tissue, robotics to enable paraplegics to walk independently, electronic diagnosis, the restocking of our antibacterial armory, widespread use of gene therapy, and the reduction of toxic chemicals to protect future health.

There is already an impressive rise in telemedicine and telehealth as well as major advances in remote robotic surgery. My dentist recently told me he was at a seminar where robotic surgery was being discussed for dental implants. Many of these changes permit patients and physicians, in the remote areas of the US, to have visual access to experts who would otherwise be unavailable to them. Holograms are sent from hospitals for review and medical recommendation.

Virtual care uses artificial intelligence to filter and flag medical information, automatically moving the most serious condition to the top for intervention. The software can detect abnormal findings quicker than those picked up, hours later, by a physician. This holds the potential for making major differences in outcomes (25).

However, electronic medicine involves a flood of paper, fax machines, privacy barriers, information repositories, and possibly superfluous data. As we move toward increased reliance on electronic medicine, there is a need to carefully weigh the risks. The first being the fact that an increase in use of health care information technology may also increase the number of errors by those using the software. Would this technology prove daunting for homebound patients? Most importantly, would not virtual care be impersonal without the human touch that so very many of us see as central to the doctor-patient relationship? Despite these Star Trek advances, there remains the specter of noncompliance. Our present medical care differs from the care in other developed nations as a result of substantially higher prices for hospitalizations, doctor's visits, prescription drugs, and inordinately high administrative costs. The US has a lower life expectancy than many other first world countries (30). The reasons for this are multivariate and complex. However, with an appreciation of the three models, we might derive a better understanding of the underlying dynamics of these statistics.

One thing remains clear. Great doctors give their patients more than their skill. In these men and women, intellect and training are reinforced by something else that escapes definition. As previously mentioned, the science of logic never made a man reason correctly. Science lays down the guidelines within which the rules of the art must fall. My hope is that the information I've provided appeals and stimulates the original and creative aspects in each of you. To make progress, even Albert Einstein had to demolish the hidden prejudices and assumptions held, knowingly and unknowingly, by his peers. To do this, he had to uncover their assumptions and expose them to realities that were not patently obvious. Can we afford to do less?

CHAPTER 3

The Psychogenic Model

This familiar model deals with the mind and mental functions after disease has been ruled out. It must, however, be kept in mind that it is impossible to separate the mind from the body as psychological symptoms affect one's physiology.

It is important to recognize and acknowledge the present and ongoing contributions of psychiatry and psychology There are scores of individuals living productive lives due to the abilities, efforts, and intelligence of the professionals in these disciplines. In spite of depression and anxiety, among other symptoms, people function, have families, and contribute to our society.

Just knowing that someone will listen in a caring manner often has a most beneficial impact on reducing the isolation and loneliness that seems to plague so many. But like any discipline, mental health treatment poses its own unique concerns. Here, too, an increased awareness of complementary views about the determinants of behavior and alternative treatment strategies can only help mental health professionals become even more effective. I believe it is helpful to develop an awareness of the history and evolution of mental health treatment, as the past often pushes its tentacles into the present, influencing our behavior without our awareness.

Early accounts of psychiatry and psychology reveal a mixed but generally ignominious history. Despite evidence to the contrary, early treatment was based upon cruel and insensitive medical therapies. Studies proving the worthlessness of the prevailing treatments were ignored and later hidden by the drug companies as they developed new pharmaceutical treatments. I strongly suggest that one read Robert Whitaker's outstanding book, *Mad in America*. This book details the history and mistreatment of the mentally ill with a focus on those diagnosed with schizophrenia. I have drawn heavily on this book with its impressive documentation.

The legacy of the past, with its negative connation of mental illness, continues to this day. Patients with a "mental problem" are often treated differently by physicians than those who present with physical concerns. Those suffering with emotional issues are prone to compound their difference by holding a negative image of themselves. They may perceive themselves as though they are not only different from but also less valued than the rest of the general population. Shame, insecurity, and self-doubt often become entrenched emotions, and this diminished self-image has a marked influence on social and occupational functioning. While the historical treatments I'll be describing also reflect the social and philosophical values of an earlier period, I will leave it up to the reader to decide for themselves how much has changed.

During the 19th century, there were two competing theories of treatments for the "insane." One approach was influenced by Philippe Pinel who, in 1793, removed the shackles from the patients at the Salpetriere and Bicetre asylums in Paris. At the same time, an ethical treatment was also being advanced by the Quakers in England. Kindness was the hallmark of their treatment. Eventually, this approach spread to America and in the asylums, patients were exposed to gardening, reading, games, in addition to opportunities for education. When trusted, patients would be permitted to stroll the grounds and even go into town. Friends Asylum in Philadelphia (today known as Friends Hospital) constantly reported that 50 percent of all admissions left cured (54). Social workers at that time were largely responsible for this moral treatment of the insane. However, the rise of this effective moral treatment threatened the physicians of that period.

It must be understood the medical approach of that time was a reflection of beliefs about man's nature. At the beginning of the

20th century, the mentally ill were seen as carriers of defective germplasms. Since these individuals often lacked the capacity for reasoned behavior, civilized society would ultimately decline. Therefore, the insane had to be cured if they were to regain their ability to reason and be productive. One approach to treatment was predicated on the belief that the patient needed to fear the omnipotence of their physician. Out of this philosophy evolved medical treatments designed to dominate and control patients. Chemicals were used to induce nausea and vomiting so the patient would not have the strength or desire to exhibit deranged behaviors. To achieve this goal, patients were, at times, subjected to starvation, excessive bleedings, and intense pain caused by rubbing caustic irritants on shaved heads. The use of physical restraints was common in addition to beatings. Dr. Benjamin Rush, the leading authority on madness in America, developed his "tranquilizer chair," which he believed aided in curing madness. Strapped in this chair, the patient was totally immobilized with their vision blocked; they were often doused with hot and cold water. It was not unusual for the individual to remain in this contraption for hours until considered tranquilized (54).

In the late 1880s, some physicians added drowning therapy to their treatments. After the patient was nearly drowned, they were resuscitated. The object of this lesson was to force the patient into taking a new start in life by leaving their disease behind. Pinel believed these remedies, advanced in medical texts, were rarely useful and frequently injurious. He expressed the opinion these approaches to treatment arose from "prejudices, hypotheses, pedantry, ignorance, and the authority of celebrated names." Unfortunately, Pinel's lessons were generally ignored.

One exception was the moral treatment of a Quaker physician, Dr. Thomas Kirkbride. In 1842, he opened a new asylum, the Pennsylvania Hospital located in West Philadelphia. At that time, it had an appealing dining area plus a game room and bowling alley. Eventually, a greenhouse and museum were added. Patients were roused at 6AM for exercise in the gymnasium. Men would wear suits with ties, and women often wore dresses. The hospital offered lectures, concerts, theatrical performances, and educational instruction in reading and sewing. Most importantly, Dr. Kirkbride taught patients that through their exercise of their free will they could choose to be sane and control or even eliminate their symptoms. Despite this approach, only some benefited. Many remained hospitalized for indeterminate periods of time and sadly became the chronic backward patients.

By the end of the 19th and beginning of the 20th century, the eugenics movement took hold in America. We witnessed the first laws for the compulsory sterilization of the mentally ill along with other "unfit" members of our society. This movement was funded by John D. Rockefeller Jr., Andrew Carnegie, and other graduates of ivy league universities.

By 1914, eugenics was taught as a science in the most prestigious of our universities. That same year, a national conference, funded by the inventor of the cereal, John Harvey Kellogg, defined a major objective of the eugenics movement. The objective was to sterilize 5.76 million Americans in order to reduce the percentage of defectives in the population to an acceptable level. Eventually, grouped with the mentally ill, were the other "unfits." These included the poor, criminals, and the mentally handicapped.

WWI gave additional impetus to the eugenics movement. Many believed the majority of American war causalities included the most fit and able of society. The implication being those who did not serve and remained at home were the unfit. Therefore, science felt an obligation to enlighten the government about the need to prevent and stop the spread of the inferior members of our culture (54). Speakers from our finest universities gave talks on the cost of taking care of defectives, the inheritance of insanity, and the low birth rates of the elite. The movement did not stop there. Articles in prominent newspapers expressed concerns about "the Jewish Problem," the dangers of "Negro-White Intermixture," and "the Pedigree of Pauper Stocks." The reader may now better understand the real reasons behind the 1924 immigration quota I wrote about earlier.

In 1929, it was reported that 85 percent of the sterilized mentally ill were either thankful for the surgery or indifferent to it. In 1935, 85 percent of all Californians favored eugenic sterilization of the mentally ill. The only ones who were not surveyed were those who had been sterilized. America's eugenic approach to social ills did have a profound influence on Nazi Germany, where eugenics was carried to terrifying extremes.

During the following years, there arose a multitude of approaches to treating and curing the mentally ill. Gynecologists claimed that hysterectomies and the removal of ovaries demonstrated improvement in more than 50 percent of insane females. Psychiatrists, influenced by new knowledge of hormonal functions, injected the mentally ill with extracts from animals' ovaries, testicles, pituitaries, and thyroids. Not surprisingly, these physicians always claimed a fair degree of success from their treatment (54).

By the 1930s, influenced by the earlier work of the psychiatrist Dr. Manfred Sakel in Vienna, insulin coma therapy came to prominence in the US. Psychiatrists eventually began using Metrazol, a drug that triggered explosive seizures. Patients would violently arch into convulsions, often causing spinal fractures, broken jaws and teeth, among other injuries. Autopsies revealed that Metrazol also caused hemorrhages in internal organs, including the brain. Like the induced insulin coma, Metrazol shock therapy required a course of treatment of 20, 30, and possibly 40 or more injections to produce a change in behavior. Metrazol injections were terrifying. Patients would often be reduced to pleading, crying, and exhibiting regressive behaviors to avoid another treatment. The majority of patients also experienced the terror of impending death in addition to the other loathsome effects from the treatment.

By 1940, electroconvulsive shock was introduced as a better way to induce longer seizures and greater amnesia. The purpose of induced amnesia through seizures was to eliminate hallucinations along with other targeted symptoms. Physicians were quite aware of the underlying brain damage that was responsible for any reduction of symptoms. It eventually became evident that electroshock's curative benefits dissipated with time, and psychosis often returned. It is interesting, for readers with a psychological background, that Lauretta Bender (of the Bender-Gestalt Test) put a toddler younger than three years of age through 20 electroconvulsive shock treatments. However, one has to view this treatment through the lens of that era.

I would be remiss if I did not mention the practice of prefrontal lobotomies. It was promulgated by early physicians, many of whom were motivated by a desire for recognition and prestige. It was not uncommon for proponents of the treatment to announce only positive outcomes. By 1937, the *New York Times* reported, "This new operation was a panacea that could relieve anxiety, depression, insomnia, suicidal ideas, delusions, hallucinations, crying spells, obsessions, panic states, along with almost all psychological problems. All one had to do was injure the frontal lobes of the brain described as a harmless procedure by the medical practitioners." By the 1940s, the medical success of lobotomies was top news, and its use exploded. More than 20,000 people had undergone the surgery by 1955. College graduates suffering from neurosis were considered good candidates. It is important to remember the beliefs physicians still held stemmed from the eugenics movement. And, the prevailing societal views at that time still reflected the opinion that those with mental illness did not have any intrinsic value. These beliefs supported and justified the need for lobotomies (54).

There were critics of the procedure who described a lobotomy as a surgically-induced childhood. Recovering patients would be given children's and infants' toys to occupy themselves. Those who had been artists or musicians became apathetic in pursuing and demonstrating their talents. A number of psychiatrists acknowledged that 25 percent of their lobotomized patients would be considered at the level of an invalid or domestic pet. Simple tasks, for many, would prove to be difficult, and sexual behavior often regressed to immature levels. Lobotomized subjects often became aggressive and inappropriate, showing no consideration for their partner. Despite these results, a significant number of physicians felt this was not really a terrible outcome for the patient.

Physicians like Dr. Walter Freeman, motivated by money and fame, vigorously promoted the merits of the transorbital lobotomy. He went on to develop what he considered a simplified operation. No longer were holes drilled in the sides of the patient's head, where he previously had inserted his scalpel. He now attacked the frontal lobes through the eye sockets. Eliminating anesthesia, he would knock the patient out with electroshock and then use an ice pick to poke a hole in the bony orbit above each eye. After the ice pick was inserted into the brain, Dr. Freeman would move behind the patient and pull up on the pick to destroy the frontal lobe fibers. He considered this a minor 20-minute operation, which did not require hospitalization or even the sterilization of the operating field. Eventually, he traveled from asylum to asylum charging 25 dollars for each procedure. He eventually used two ice picks to simultaneously pierce both eyes (54).

Between the 1930s and the 1970s, the US performed between 40,000 to 50,000 lobotomies, more than any other country in the world. The Stockton State Hospital in California lobotomized 232 patients. This fortunately ended in 1954 when 125 patients died from the surgery and others suffered lasting and terrible side effects. Readers may remember President John F. Kennedy's sister, Rosemary, the oldest daughter of the Kennedy family, who had a lobotomy at age 23. This resulted in her inability to ever walk or speak again. In spite of terrible outcomes, Dr. Freeman's lobotomies were described by newspapers as "easier than curing a toothache." Again, we are forced to ask whose good was really being served by these surgeries. In spite of the overwhelming evidence, the influence of eugenics continued. Insulin comas, electroshock therapy, and brain-damaging lobotomies remained prominent treatments in asylum medicine until the mid-20th century.

The modern era of medical treatments for schizophrenia began in May 1954 when Smith, Kline & French (SKF) introduced the first antipsychotic drug, chlorpromazine sold as Thorazine. SKF, along with the press, advertised Thorazine as a medication that represented one of the most significant advances in the history of psychiatry. Suddenly, it was possible for the family physician to treat mental illness in their offices. Nothing was mentioned by drug companies at the time about multiple studies revealing the drug caused Parkinson's symptoms and lethargy. Additional reviews from medical researchers on the value of this drug were mixed. Some physicians felt its only value was to make hospital patients easier to manage while others hoped it would replace hospital care.

Despite this uncertainty, the power and influence of the pharmaceutical companies escalated. SKF charged six times what the inventors of chlorpromazine in France could charge. Thorazine initially cost SKF $350,000 and in a short time its revenues skyrocketed into the hundreds of millions. Ongoing studies that revealed the drug made patients immobile, wax-like, and emotionally indifferent continued to be ignored.

The goal of the National Institute of Mental Health (NIMH) was to reduce, even eliminate, the burden of the cost of public mental hospitals. Disregarding the negative effects of Thorazine, NIMH felt there was enough scientific rationale for discharging patients into the community thanks to this medication (54).

Thorazine was not considered a cure for schizophrenia, as multiple researchers understood the drug (now classified as a neuroleptic) achieved its effects by hindering brain function and did not normalize brain chemistry. It inhibited the activity of the neurotransmitter dopamine, which caused the Parkinson's symptoms when high doses of this medication were administered.

The next drugs targeted for schizophrenia included Prolixin and Haldol, which were 50 times more potent than Thorazine. These drugs were developed by Squibb and Janssen pharmaceutical companies. Squibb's injectable formulation of Prolixin shut down dopaminergic pathways so rapidly it was often described as "instant Parkinson's." By the middle of the 1980s, patients were discharged from hospitals on inordinately high doses of these neuroleptics with the corresponding negative side effects like those of severe Parkinson's disease. As usual, the harm done was borne by the patient. The high-dose patient was also found to suffer with increased depression, anxiety, motor retardation, and other negative side effects. When patients on heavy doses did relapse, they often became severely ill. A daily dose of 20 milligrams of Haldol, which was the standard in the 1980s, caused significant deterioration in the emotional response and social functioning of patients (54).

In 1969, the Soviets began using neuroleptics for their negative side effects to punish dissidents. We could not readily condemn the Russians as we were diagnosing more people with schizophrenia than all other developed countries. This diagnosis was not free from racial, political, or class bias. In 1958, the first African American to apply to the University of Mississippi, Clennon King, was admitted to a state mental hospital. Obviously, he had to be "out of touch with reality" if he thought he could get into Ole Miss. In the early 1970s, US institutions were routinely using neuroleptics to quiet the mentally retarded, the elderly, and the juvenile delinquents.

Newer drugs have since been developed, most notably atypical antipsychotics which have received some acclaim. However, the research is plagued with deception, terrible controls, poor design, and ulterior financial motives. Fraud continues to this day in the marketing of new pharmaceuticals. The biggest question is how these new drugs will affect patients' lives in the long term. After studying the older drugs, the World Health Organization concluded they ultimately "led to an increase in chronic illness and limited the possibility of recovery." In his epilogue, Robert Whitaker concluded that "in 1998, British investigators reviewed the published results of 2,000 clinical trials of neuroleptics over the past 50 years and found that only one in 25 studies even bothered to assess daily living activities or social functioning. The investigations repeatedly looked at whether the drugs knocked down the visible symptoms of psychosis and ignored what was really happening to the patient as people." While medications do have a major role in treating mental illness, they must be used with wisdom and respect for the individual who bears the consequence of using any medication. This makes it even more important for treating professionals to consider options to alleviate suffering, and I again encourage the reader to question who really benefits from new treatments.

A 2005 study conducted to investigate the last 50 years of treatment for mental illness showed a dramatic increase of the mentally ill in the US. Since 1955, there was a fivefold increase in severe mental illness. That was the year Thorazine was introduced as psychiatry's first wonder drug. However, by 1987, mental illness nearly doubled. A careful review of nearly 6 million Americans disabled by mental illness in 2005 revealed that it was due to a drug-based paradigm of care. The drugs being used at that time increased the likelihood that the treated person would become chronically ill with more severe psychiatric symptoms (54).

Current studies are concerned about how newer drugs will affect patients' lives over longer periods of time. The older antipsychotics or neuroleptics led to an increase in chronic illness and limited the possibility of recovery. One neurologist told me that the antipsychotics changed receptor sites in the brain, and when the brain adapted to these changes it required ever increasing amounts of the drug to control the behavior for which it was initially given. This helps to explain why physicians are frequently obligated to increase the doses of neuroleptics to manage symptoms (55).

With respect to schizophrenia, one has to question whether it is a discrete illness. The new Diagnostic and Statistical Manual of Mental Disorders (DSM-5) represents a sincere attempt to clear up the issues of diagnosis, but the reliability of the diagnosis is the problem and new names do not constitute knowledge.

As previously mentioned, I had been an undergraduate research assistant assigned to Haverford State Hospital in Haverford, Pennsylvania. Watching television one evening, I was surprised to see two patients from the alcoholic unit in a 30-minute program about how they benefited from psychiatric treatment with LSD—lysergic acid diethylamide. I was not aware that a male and female from my unit had been treated with this psychedelic drug. All I knew about LSD was that the actor Cary Grant had taken this drug as part of his psychotherapy. Both Grant and the pharmaceutical company Sandoz claimed LSD treatments shortened the need for extensive therapy sessions and brought successful treatment outcomes. The TV program ended on the most positive of notes. I clearly remember the final scene where these two individuals were romping through sunlit fields; the world was bright and the future hopeful. The reality was quite different, as I later discovered. I learned that both the man and the woman had been readmitted for suicidal and homicidal tendencies. It was known that LSD produced psychological effects that included an altered awareness of one's surroundings as well as changes in perception, feelings, and sensations. I personally witnessed a terrified student who perceived his mind was irretrievably leaving his body after taking LSD. For some, LSD abuse resulted in an irreversible psychosis. I was shocked there was never a follow-up to the initial TV show that showed the dangers of using this psychedelic. What I came to realize was that the show was basically a 30-minute commercial for LSD, and the sale of the drug was apparently more important than the consequences for patients.

On another occasion, while providing services in the psychiatric unit of Abington Hospital, I was asked to see a man who had multiple in-patient admissions for suicide attempts. The patient, an artist, worked in a factory making electrical components.

When he had enough money saved, he travelled the world to take photographs and then returned to his studio to paint. However, over a 14-year period, he made multiple suicide attempts after repeatedly scratching his body and face until they were almost shredded. Following my completed evaluation, I asked him if behavioral therapy had ever been suggested during his years of treatment. He answered no and asked me for more information. Because he was not my patient, I told him I would make the suggestion to his psychiatrist. A few days later, I received a call from his physician, who asked if we might co-treat the patient. Since we took different approaches to treatment, I told him I was not comfortable with his suggestion and that I preferred to treat alone. Days later, the psychiatrist again phoned and indicated I could see his patient for seven visits only.

I saw this gentleman at my office and, as was my general approach, I gave him homework. By homework, I mean behaviors and techniques that the patient could utilize between visits. I detailed a behavioral extinction program that permitted the patient to scratch all he wanted but only in certain locations, both at home and work. He returned a second week and we tweaked the program where necessary. The third week, he arrived wearing short sleeves and sat across from me. Arms folded, he asked: "Do you see anything different about me?" I looked at him and indicated I did not. He pointed to his bare arm and said, "I have hair on my arm for the first time in 14 years." There was no need to see him for the additional treatments, and he returned to his psychiatrist. Did I cure him? I never knew all of his problems, but

I did know he was a complex patient. Our contract was simply to control the scratching and this he did.

I believe in trying to help the patient become independent of the therapist by offering them strategies commensurate with their capacities. The aim of each strategy is to give the patient an experience of some improvement as the result of their own efforts. To see a patient one hour each week and expect to change their behavior is unrealistic and unfair. In life, do we not, in some sense, have to become our own "therapist"? So why not make these lessons part of the treatment approach early in therapy, as long as the safety and well-being of the patient are the first considerations? I maintain the real therapy begins when the patient leaves the office and utilizes some of their newly acquired skills. However, the patient is free to phone me between visits as often as they need. My responsibility does not end when they leave my office.

My wife is also a psychologist specializing in neonatal development and problems associated with adoptions, foreign and domestic. Because we are both in the same department of psychiatry, we went to meet the newly appointed department chairman, introduce ourselves, and wish her well. We spoke with her awhile and let her know we had been in her department for 25 years. I pointed out that since our inpatients remained for a relatively short time and the readmission rates were quite high, we had an obligation to teach the patients coping strategies that they might use to help themselves after discharge from our unit. Before waiting to even hear what I had in mind, she replied, "No, our job is to treat and street. The rest is someone else's responsibility." With this attitude, could she ever be effective or respected by the hospital staff? Even more importantly, her attitude had to be communicated to all her staff along with the patients. I know it ultimately harmed both. We should be aware that the language we use, verbal and nonverbal, determines the message we impart to others.

Therapy, like all scientific disciplines, has its own language. To become proficient in a particular science, one must learn the language of that science. If a physicist mentioned relativity, quarks, or singularities, other physicists would immediately know what he was talking about. We code a tremendous amount of information with words.

A perfect example is the legacy of Sigmund Freud. While he did not endow us with medications, he had a tremendous impact on the language of psychiatry and psychology. Freud's life spanned one of the most creative periods in the history of science. Darwin published the *On the Origin of Species*, making man a legitimate object of scientific study. Fechner founded the science of psychology. There were also the contributions from Pasteur, Koch, Mendel, the Curies, and Helmholtz, who formulated the principle of the conservation of energy. In this stimulating atmosphere, Freud, an Austrian physician, initially specialized in physiology and neurology. His early contributions included an influential paper on aphasia and research on cerebral palsy. For two years, he was a proponent and user of cocaine as a stimulant and analgesic; he also advocated it for depression. His advocacy ended as a result of the death of his friend Ernst Fleischl-Marxow and Freud's own untoward reactions to the drug. Because of the Nazis, Freud left Austria for England in 1938 and died in 1939. Four of his elderly sisters would later die in concentration camps (27).

Freud eventually devoted his efforts to the development of psychoanalysis. He believed there were dynamic forces causing transformations and exchanges of energy within the personality. These forces were responsible for creating the abnormal symptoms that were outside of conscious awareness. Essentially, the human being is an energy-consuming system. We derive our energy from food. It takes energy to think, feel, see, touch, smell, and to live and deal with our emotions. If we use our limited energy to deal with psychic conflicts, we may then develop neurotic symptoms like anxiety and depression.

Most have heard of the id, ego, and superego. Freud believed a person's behavior was the result of the interaction of these three systems. Simply stated, the id operates according to the pleasure principle. The pleasure principle names the tendency to avoid pain and seek pleasure. The ego is necessary because it permits the organism to transact with the objective world of reality in order to meet its needs. The superego represents our conscience pushing us toward the ideal—striving for perfection. Unfortunately, we often use and treat these three terms as though they were ghostly realities.

The defense mechanisms discovered by Freud have a marked influence on the thinking and language of psychiatry and psychology. These mechanisms protect us from anxiety or guilt, and if they are truly working, they function beyond our conscious control. Freud considered these mechanisms to be natural and normal. However, if overused, defense mechanisms could give rise to neuroses, which are evidenced by symptoms including anxiety states, phobias, obsessions, and hysteria.

The following defense mechanisms are commonly used as a part of our language. **Regression** names a movement back in psychological time that can occur when individuals are faced with overwhelming stress. The term describes behavior that appears somewhat primitive. A common example is that of a young toddler who returns to bed-wetting or to thumb-sucking when a new sibling arrives home with mom from the hospital. The mechanism of **displacement** refers to the satisfaction of an impulse like aggression through the use of a substitute object. An example might involve one's having a bad day at work and hating the boss, only to arrive home and direct the anger at a spouse or the household cat. **Projection** is a defense mechanism used to attribute our own unacceptable thoughts, feelings, and motivations to another person. **Repression** is defined as a function of the ego that blocks certain thoughts from becoming conscious. If an unacceptable thought is truly repressed, we will not be able to recall it. **Denial** blocks external events from our awareness. The last defense mechanism I will mention is **sublimation**, which consists in the satisfaction of an impulse using a substitute object in a socially appropriate way. It is important to remember that these mechanisms operate beyond our conscious awareness.

We also use the terms unconscious or subconscious to refer to quality of mind and mental states. Many of us have said, "he's anal" or talked about a Freudian slip. Clearly, Freud has shaped our language in a way that allows us to describe personality and behavior with greater ease. It also is interesting to note that some of the language medicine uses still echoes the continued use of Pythagorean metaphors borrowed from music. These include tone, tonic, well-tempered, and temperance, to name a few. Pythagoreans regarded the body as a kind of musical instrument where each string must have the correct balance between opposites such as high and low, hot and cold, and wet and dry (32).

Beyond the influence on language, Freudians and psychoanalytic theory have profoundly shaped the treatment of hospital patients. By the mid 1950s, half of all hospital patients in the US were diagnosed with mental disorders. Psychoanalysis helped move patients from the hospital and the asylum to the office with its talk therapy. However, the emphasis psychoanalysis places on childhood sexuality among other theoretical tenets makes it a controversial discipline. Its validity as a science remains open to question even now. Outcome studies of long-term psychoanalysis suggest it may not only be ineffective but might possibly have negative effects.

Before moving on to additional research, I want to discuss psychological testing. Testing is to psychologists what prescribing medication is to psychiatrists. In graduate school, one is required to administer psychological tests as a professional rite of passage. There are a multitude of instruments to assess things like personality, achievement, and brain damage, to name but a very few. A major assessment with which readers will be familiar is the IQ test. I was working part time as a welder and needed subjects for the IQ test. Fortunately, I had a ready and willing population. During breaks or on my lunch hour, I would sit on an I-beam and test the other welders along with additional willing subjects.

Test results revealed that many would have done well in college or any other endeavor. Their life went in one direction and mine in another. My last subject was a 19-year-old young man who had the dreadful job of spray painting the steel we had just finished welding. He would spray while the rest of us hid so as not to get the overspray of the lead paint on us. I finished his IQ test and after scoring found he had an IQ in the low 70s. This score, according to the "normal curve" suggested he was functioning in the "borderline retarded range." Yet this teenager drove his own car, had an apartment, and was working full time. However, in our classes we were taught this low score would have mitigated against his level of functioning. This young man's life, in addition to other experiences of his, made me realize that a score or number alone reveals next to nothing about the individual. In school, I am sure this young painter would have been labeled and treated as though he had limited abilities to learn and function. Worse still, our behavior toward him could have convinced him of his own limited potential and value.

With continued practice, I came to understand the "normal curve" is not an icon but a tool used to gather a small piece of data. It is not a description of a person's ability or worth. We all live in a social system with multiple and varied experiences shaping our actions and our capacity to function. Those of us who are privileged to work with or treat others are obligated to look beyond single measures in which experts sometimes vest in inordinate amount of power. One must refrain from making a prophecy with limited information.

Mental health providers have always been plagued with the issue of diagnosis. Dr. Morton Kramer's paper "A Cross-National Study of Diagnosis" indicated that "the diagnosis which a given individual receives is indicative of or reflective of: the psychiatric school; the ethnic background and the age of the diagnostician." Canadian psychiatrist Dr. Heinz Lehmann felt that psychiatric diagnosis "has deteriorated from being a fine and useful craft into an ill-regulated, superficial, unconvincing, and therefore often useless procedure." Dr. David Rosenhan, a psychology professor at Stanford University, attempted to test Dr. Lehman's point. He and seven other people went to 12 different mental hospitals and presented with fake symptoms. These included hearing fake voices that said things like "thud," "empty," or "hollow." Otherwise, they presented their social behaviors as normal. All of these "pseudo-patients" were admitted as inpatients and diagnosed with schizophrenia. The eight patients were given 2,100 neuroleptic pills that they flushed down the toilet. Only the other patients noticed that the eight pseudo-patients were not ill.

The study was then run in reverse. Dr. Rosenhan told a prestigious teaching hospital that during the next 90 days, pseudo-patients would try to be admitted. In reality, no one made any attempt at admission during this phase. However, over the course of the next 90-day period, this hospital admitted 193 psychiatric patients and identified 41 as pseudo-patients. His conclusion was that "we have known for a long time that diagnoses are often not useful or reliable, but we nevertheless continue to use them." Rosenhan wrote in *Science*, "We now know that we cannot distinguish sanity from insanity" (54).

The diagnosis of mental illness in African Americans has a terribly shameful history. Black males are disproportionately diagnosed in the more severe and dangerous categories. Historically, the poor too have been overly represented among the insane. I have observed that diagnoses fluctuate in popularity as times change. A number of years ago, the diagnosis of multiple personality disorder was in vogue. During one of my hospital-based monthly conferences, a psychiatrist said he was treating 12 patients with this disorder. I along with the psychiatrists in attendance looked in disbelief. In almost 50 years of practice, I believe I have seen only one patient with the full symptom complex associated with a true multiple personality disorder. I have treated patients who share some similar traits, and it is distinctly possible I missed the proper diagnosis in some of these cases. I honestly believe that I never saw a pure *Three Faces of Eve* patient as depicted in the 1957 film. Perhaps others have had different experiences with this multiple personality disorder.

Presently, it appears, the diagnosis of bipolar disorder is quite common. Diagnosis also varies with location (49). If I were to exhibit psychotic-like symptoms in our country, I would stand a 33 percent chance of being classified as a schizophrenic. I might also have been diagnosed with a psychotic-depressive reaction, a category almost nonexistent in England and Wales. In middle age, the ratio of British to American patients diagnosed as manic-depressives is 22 to 1, although this appears to be changing.

It is important to understand the term diagnosis. This word implies how the person's symptoms relate to a specific disease in clinical medicine. While psychiatry may use the same term, it really reflects a system for classifying people's complaints. It is a descriptive term for the symptoms but not their causes, as is the case in medicine. The problem in psychiatry and psychology lies in the agreement of different doctors about a patient's diagnosis or classification. An excellent review in "The Reliability of Psychiatric Diagnosis Revisited" concluded after looking at three generations up to the present, "that the reliability of psychiatric diagnosis among practicing clinicians is still poor" (1).

As previously mentioned, I had been on the staff of a very large medical hospital in the inpatient unit of the Department of Psychiatry. One day, I was asked by the department chairman to see one of his patients for diagnostic testing. The department chairman was an affable gentleman who was generally respected by his staff of psychiatrists. I completed my evaluation and in chatting with the patient, I asked how long he had been in treatment with the department's chairman. He replied that it had been 25 years, adding that he thought he was getting better. I was taken aback as I thought, "after 25 years, you still did not have a diagnosis and now you want one? What were you treating him for all this time?" Effective treatment in every medical field including psychiatry and psychology begins with a reasonably accurate diagnosis. The diagnosis is a description of the behavior targeted for change.

The ability for an accurate mental health diagnosis, while always of major significance, has become critical to the well-being of our nation. In 1966, Charles Whitman climbed the clock tower of the University of Texas and used a rifle to kill 13 and wound 30 students. We might not remember that horrific nightmare, but we likely remember Columbine, Sandy Hook, Aurora, Orlando, and Parkland. We should not forget the tragedies reported every day throughout the US stemming from the increasing number of neighborhood shootings. Yet our legislators, the savants who guide and protect us, offer vapid suggestions as solutions. They refuse to pass federal gun laws that block the sale of AR-15s. They are at the very least naïve and often exhibit spineless behavior. There is no excuse for those who will not even take the time to learn that their recommendations are meaningless solutions or worse. I am reminded of Thomas Henry Huxley's quote as it relates to stopping the slaughter of innocents, "Many a beautiful theory was killed by an ugly fact." There is continued resistance to the implementation of existing technology that would permit the gun owner to be the sole individual capable to firing his or her weapon. However, keeping guns out of the hands of the "mentally ill" is still a popular refrain. No one would disagree but, as we have seen, we do not have a real ability to identify the mentally ill. Do we use medical records if someone has seen a psychiatrist or psychologist? If you were to go to your physician because you suspected a broken arm, had it x-rayed, and it was negative, the physician would receive payment from your insurance carrier for this negative result. If you saw a psychologist for a minor complaint and a bill was submitted, the therapist would not receive payment unless a mental issue was diagnosed. Even the most minor diagnosis would probably go in your medical file somewhere.

It seems clear that mental illness is difficult and often impossible to determine unless one is blatantly psychotic. A frequent recommendation involves allocating more money for mental health treatment. While money may be somewhat helpful, it is hardly a solution. Research has established that psychiatry and psychology are ineffective in reaching a consensus on diagnoses. Though there are exceptions, this means we are not effective enough at identifying those with mental illness much less those who will commit these atrocities (43). This is true regardless of the amount of money spent to ease the conscience of our legislators and placate those of us who remain outraged and insulted, and feel impotent. If the pharmaceutical firms put money before health, why should we be surprised that gun manufacturers behave in the same manner?

There are competent clinicians with outstanding skills, but we need more. It is vital that we have improved training dealing with the multiple reasons for mental illness as well as alternative strategies for treatment. We can no longer rely on toilet-trained approaches to treatment and outdated theories of causality for mental aberrations. Refer back to the "enabler model," developed by Dr. Robert Kleiner, which did not depend on M.D.s or Ph.D.s, but looked instead to our social system for new and improvised treatment strategies. The standard strategies have not worked, and we really don't require more shootings to prove it. In the next chapter, I hope to provide a greater understanding of this problem and consider it from different perspectives. If we are ever to increase our ability to be more generative with our solutions to social issues, we must be receptive to correcting our thinking.

I was consulted to see a patient who was living independently in a life care facility. This woman, in her mid-80s, was suffering from visual hallucinations and was being considered for transfer to a psychiatric facility. While looking in the mirror, she also saw a little girl who she would try to feed. When I stood next to the woman and we both looked into the mirror, she saw the two of us as well as the small child. She would take some of her lunch and try to shove it into the mirror to feed the girl. Apart from these hallucinations, the resident was functioning independently. In an attempt to stop the visual hallucination, the staff covered the large bathroom mirror. When I stood next to the woman, with the mirror now covered, she would take the half of her sandwich and try to shove it into the plaster wall next to the covered mirror. She remained convinced the child was still there. When I asked about her vision, I was told she had age-related macular degeneration. I suspected this was the explanation for her visual disturbance and believed she was suffering from Charles Bonnet syndrome. Visual hallucinations are characteristic of this disorder and often feature young children. I phoned her ophthalmologist, explained my observations, and he agreed to take care of his patient. As a mental health professional, it is essential that we consider alternative possibilities before reaching a conclusion about an individual's behavior.

While working in the same facility, I had to pass through the locked dementia unit to go to the administrative offices on the fourth floor. As I passed by the lunchroom, I saw and heard a patient screaming uncontrollably. This was, of course, upsetting the rest of the residents eating lunch. The nurse in charge went to her medication cart for a neuroleptic that was ordered to control this behavior. I was unfamiliar with the patient but knew the nurse and requested she hold the medication. I went over to the woman and asked, "Would you do me a favor and dance with me?" She stopped screaming, and we danced for 30 seconds near her lunch table. That was the end of her outbursts; no medication was necessary and she along with the other residents seemed to enjoy the brief interlude. We often forget that demented patients retain motor memories; they can, as in this example, dance but they're also able to remember the "oldies" along with other long-term memories. Again, it's the model you have in your head. The screaming was seen and heard in a medical setting and the ready solution was medication, but it was not the only solution. A small change in thinking can have a major change in behavior. For example, if you tell an Alzheimer's patient not to do something, odds are they will do it. Still, it is more effective if you ask them to do something.

Relatively recent research has revealed that your gut is a sophisticated neural network that transmits messages to your head; bacteria in the gut communicates with the brain via the vagus nerve. Gut bacteria both produce and respond to the same neurochemicals such as GABA, serotonin, norepinephrine, dopamine, acetylcholine, and melatonin that the brain uses to regulate mood and cognition. It is, however, a two-way street and psychological stress can suppress beneficial bacteria. Some psychiatrists now suggest using probiotics to treat depression. The human microbiome is, however, quite complex and the science of probiotics is still quite new. The use of these nutrients should be under the direction of a functional medicine physician or another expert. A good national database for more than 8,000 foods is: http://ndb.nal.usda.gov/.

The implication here is that, to fully understand our emotions and behavior, we may also need to study the gut as much as the brain. When I see a patient in the medical center and I know there is a significant problem in the stomach, I will always ask the psychiatrist to consider using an antidepressant. The reason is that problems in the gut generate the same neuropeptides that are found with depression in the brain (10). This reflects an additional approach to the understanding of the mind-body connection. The beauty of holding different models is that it enables one to see a problem from multiple viewpoints. This increases your potential to correctly understand and, when necessary, effectively intervene.

Suicide remains a significant problem, and I believe it is not yet well understood. We will look at this behavior in greater detail in the following chapter. Antidepressants seem to have more benefit for those who were suffering from major depression but only in the short-term. It is unclear how well antidepressants work with milder depression, even if the person has been on these medications for months or years. It is also possible that some of the benefit from these medications may be due to the placebo effect. We are aware that virtually all drugs work at least in part via the placebo effect and more so with antidepressants (9).

Outcome studies on the efficacy of medications is always open to questioning. Research has shown antipsychotics are relatively useless against certain behaviors associated with Alzheimer's disease. Alzheimer's patients given Zyprexa, Seroquel, or Risperdal for eight weeks fared no better than those given a placebo. Why do we then use these drugs? While they may serve as a quick fix in the absence of alternatives, they may also reflect incomplete knowledge about their effects on the geriatric population. The criteria to evaluate the effectiveness of any treatment for mental illness should reside with the patient. Does the patient feel he or she is better? Do they think more clearly? Are they satisfied with their lives after treatment? Are they less depressed, less anxious and, with more serious illnesses, have the hallucinations disappeared?

Presently, the best predictor for patients to be readmitted to a mental hospital is the number of previous admissions of that patient. This clearly indicates that more research is needed in the entire field of mental health. Unbiased research will not be easy. We have seen how pharmaceutical greed influenced the outcomes of drug studies. However, there are even more subtle factors at work when one conducts research.

Robert Rosenthal, the author of *Pygmalion in the Classroom,* feels the demand characteristics of experiments influences outcomes. Prior to writing his book on how teachers' expectations determined students' performances, he did work with rats. He took a group of identical rats, labelling one group smart and the other dumb. Smart rats learned to run the mazes in the experiment, while the dumb rats never learned the maze. In the middle of the night, Rosenthal switched the labels and the formally dumb rats, now labeled smart, learned the new mazes, while the dumb rats, formerly labelled smart, never learned them. Many felt his work in the lab and in the classroom cast a pall over 50 years of psychological testing.

Experimenter bias is ubiquitous and has to be guarded against. We need psychiatrists and psychologists, as they are presently our first line of help for mental problems. These professionals do the best they can in a social system that often underestimates the difficulties in treating serious intra- and interpersonal problems. Those who hold the psychogenic view must remember it reflects a way of asking questions, and the answers they receive influence their understanding and often their treatment approaches. These answers are not necessarily synonymous with truth, which reinforces the need for and benefit of holding multiple models.

It is terribly upsetting to read about the epidemiology of teen suicide. Prevention of suicide, despite antidepressant treatment, continues to be a significant social problem as evidenced by the increase in self-destructive behaviors. According to the Centers for Disease Control, the World Health Organization, and the American Foundation for Suicide Prevention, suicide is the 10th leading cause of death in the US. Each year, 44,965 Americans die by suicide, and for every suicide it is estimated there are 25 attempts. Consequently, the rate of suicide is under-reported. How many automobile accidents are really suicide attempts? If a person attempts suicide but is only injured and then later dies from the illness or injury, the death may not be reported as a suicide. On average, there are 123 suicides per day and in 2016, firearms accounted for 51 percent of these deaths. The statistics may vary with the reporting agency, but suicide occurs in all age populations, starting most often from 10 years old and increasing as the population ages (46). For some individuals, antidepressants have demonstrated some benefit when coupled with cognitive behavioral therapy. Chapter 4 opens another perspective with the hope of being able to shed additional light on this serious problem.

Again, I repeatedly emphasize the need for the reader to embrace the opportunity to hold alternative models in order to recognize and appreciate the many determinants impacting our lives. When trying to understand an event, remember that truth simplifies, clarifies, and edifies. During the first part of the last century, physicists were determined to measure the ether wind that, they believed, surrounded the earth and through which light was thought to travel. When they were unable to do so, they did not abandon science; instead, they corrected their language and abandoned the notion of the ether.

The human brain has 100 billion nerve cells with 100 trillion synapses; there are no two brains alike. But then all behavior is not determined by our internal anatomy, physiology, or psychology. This is the subject matter in the next chapter.

CHAPTER 4

The Sociogenic Model

This model is the one least understood and may be challenging to integrate into our customary ways of understanding behavior. However, I believe this model holds a great explanatory potential as it pushes us to investigate individuals within their social system. Social systems appear to be ubiquitous, appearing in 15 million species down to the spiders. Interactions between members is considered to be of paramount importance, and language is seen as an infra-communicational system. The word "sociogenic" refers to nonverbal communication within social systems, carrying a marked influence on behavior. The reader had a sample in the introduction when I asked the question,

"Who taught you to blush?" The power of the placebo is another example of nonverbal communication. We could also consider how much an infant learns about their world prior to their use of language.

In the 1940s, perfume companies provided University of Pennsylvania freshman women with a full pint of their favorite perfume for the purpose of a study. The companies measured evaporation rates, and the women in the study were asked about their use of perfume, as it related to their dating interests. How much perfume did they, for example, use when they were looking for a date, had a boyfriend, or were not interested in dating? What would be your guess as to the results of their investigations? One clue is that the perfume companies never published the results, but the anthropologists did.

The results revealed that when a woman was not interested in finding anyone special or interested in dating at all, she used the most perfume. If a student had or found a boyfriend, the least amount or no perfume was used. The anthropologists concluded that underarm hairs signal natural body attractants. Excessive perfume blocked these attraction signals, communicating a lack of interest in the opposite sex. However, not using perfume permitted the release of these signals and an attraction was communicated.

What does an infant smell like? To me, a new grandfather, there is no sweeter smell. For those who experience a close relationship with another, have you, at times, not experienced their natural fragrance? When Dr. Ray Birdwhistell published these results, he received samples of families' secret perfumes. An analysis of these samples revealed one common ingredient: vanilla extract. What does the smell of vanilla conjure up for most of us? Today, I am sure the explanation would include pheromones. This study has frequently been cited to illustrate the influence and importance of nonverbal communication (6).

I had made an earlier mention of the privilege of studying with Dr. Ray Birdwhistell at the University of Pennsylvania's Annenberg School for Communication. He had previously developed the science of kinesics, put forth in the best-selling book *Kinesics and Context* (3). During WWII, Dr. Birdwhistell first became interested in nonverbal communication and came to believe that it was fundamental for the transmission of cultural information. While in the service, he observed that a salute by a private in the US Army could be performed in a manner which could satisfy, please, or enrage the most demanding officer. By shifts in stance, facial expression, and changes in the velocity and duration of the movement, one could dignify, ridicule, demean, seduce, insult, or promote an individual. Birdwhistell saw similarities between gestures and "stem forms in language." By this, he meant there was, in body motion, behavioral shapes which were direct analogs to linguistic forms. Our bodies have virtually unlimited positional changes in muscular and skeletal forms that can vary in intensity and duration. Consequently, all members of every social system have tremendous capacity for nonverbal communication. This capacity makes it easier for us to contribute to the understanding of our community or social system than if we were a species with a single channel of communication—language. Other species without language must do this if they are to successfully produce offspring. In short, human communication is not simply a matter of words spoken, and meaning is not a simple quantity carried by particular words and sentences. Everything we don't know how to say must be conveyed by other aspects of our communication system (4).

The implication from the above brief description is that man has survived, because he could respond to information before he could verbalize it. These nonverbal capacities serve an adaptive function for the members of all social systems. Individuals in every society are interrelated and interdependent, as no one member has all the information in their culture. Rather, information is something in which all members partake; when shared, often without conscious awareness, it shapes our actions in positive or negative ways (5). While Dr. Birdwhistell is best known for inventing kinesics, he helped establish the underpinnings of language and social interaction research (7).

The three models presented provide multiple vantage points from which to better understand and, when necessary, challenge time-honored assumptions about human interactions. Holding multiple views greatly enhances our ability to introspect about our own beliefs. Thinking about a particular problem or behavior from multiple perspectives is challenging, rewarding, and essential for personal and professional growth. In what follows, I will consider the power of nonverbal communication for envisaging some of these problems and behaviors differently.

An interesting phenomenon is the Couvade syndrome, also called sympathetic pregnancy. The term originates from the behavior found in certain primitive tribes. When a woman is pregnant and a man wishes to establish his paternity, he develops symptoms typically associated with pregnancy. The expectant father may take to his bed for nine months with labor pains, morning nausea, and even weight gain. After the birth, the father responds as though he had never been ill.

Although many cases have been reported in the literature, I have only seen one case myself. It happened to my neighbor when his wife became pregnant. The husband developed labor pains, gained weight, experienced morning nausea, and exhibited particular food cravings. While this is an example of nonverbal communication, experts are divided on whether it is due to psychological or biological factors. Studies have shown the male partner living with a pregnant woman will experience hormonal shifts in his prolactin, cortisol, estradiol, and testosterone levels starting at the end of the first trimester and continuing through several weeks postpartum (14). These chemical changes in the male are clearly communicated without language.

In England in the 1930s and 1940s, there were small birds known as tits. These birds learned to take the paper lids off of milk bottles that were delivered to homes and drink the cream. Eventually, the lids had to be changed, but before that occurred, ethologists took the eggs out of the nest of mature tits and hatched them far from all adult birds. When the hatchlings matured, they were born with the knowledge and ability to fly to and open the lids of the milk bottles. How this behavior is understood will depend on your models of questioning and understanding. Is this an example of nonverbal communication and its influence on the genetic pool of these birds? I will leave the answer to the reader's investigation and cogitation.

A well published study involving nonverbal communication occurred in the women's freshman dormitories at the University of Pennsylvania. When these women started college, their menstrual cycles occurred randomly during the calendar month. By mid-semester, the women tended to have their menses around the same time. This phenomenon has also been observed in women's prisons, long-term care mental hospitals, and even in neighborhoods where women have almost no contact with one another. Some believe that women in close-knit groups are unconsciously pushing and pulling on one another's cycles, mediated by pheromones. It is also known that the communication through pheromones is not something that occurs solely between individuals, but also within the same female. Studies support the findings that a woman's sexual responsivity is first triggered by visual stimuli and followed by her body's own secretion of pheromones. Women unconsciously smell pheromones, which act as a determinant of sexual feelings. We will look at an additional explanation to understand the tendency of women to cycle together (6).

I'm originally from Philadelphia and often frequented Roosevelt Boulevard, a major and terribly fast-moving thoroughfare, where automobile accidents are commonplace. In one dangerous intersection, the city placed signs that read something like: "This intersection is the highest accident area in Philadelphia." The sign had a very short life and was removed from the intersection, as the number of accidents only increased. For some, the sign appeared to offer an excuse for where they had their accident.

Franz Boas, considered the "Father of American Anthropology," was born in Germany in 1858. He studied tribal peoples and cultures from all over the world and eventually made anthropology his life's work. Dr. Boas made a study of morphological attributes as they were influenced by environmental changes. He posed the following question. If a married couple from Europe, whose head shapes were oval, immigrated to the US and had a child, what would be the head shape of their offspring? Genetics would suggest the child would probably have an oval head shape like those of the parents. However, Boas found the head would take on the shape of the dominant culture in which the child was raised. His investigations suggested this hereditary marker of race was, in fact, sensitive to environmental change within a single generation. To Boas, even high heritability may not be as important as the culture in which the child is raised (23).

Boas introduced the tenets of cultural relativism and exhibited tireless efforts to end bigotry and oppression. He attacked the beliefs of white supremacy by showing with solid evidence that there was no innate racial inheritance guaranteeing the white man's natural right to rule. It is interesting to read a few of his quotes. "If we were to select the most intelligent, imaginative, energetic, and emotionally stable third of mankind, all races would be present." "The existence of any pure race with special endowments is a myth, as is the belief that there are races all of whose members are foredoomed to eternal inferiority." With this model, Boas challenged many prevailing ideas about human biology and race.

Additional data, helping us to understand the shift in head shapes, comes from forensic pathologists. Their investigations suggest they are able, from examining aspects of the skulls, to determine the part of the US in which the individual lived. Bone changes in the face can be seen as a result of our having regional accents acquired in a particular culture during our formative years. Different models yield contrasting information.

We have been looking at events at a macro level, but it is also interesting to consider them at the micro level. Let us assume that one member of a pair of entangled subatomic particles flies off and is separated from the other particle by an infinite distance. However, if something changes the direction and momentum of one of the particles, the effect on the other particle is instantaneous and similar. This is known as the Einstein-Podolsky-Rosen paradox. Einstein called it, "Spooky action at a distance" (22). This phenomenon helped provide the impetus for investigating quantum information, a science that has enriched our lives. It is obvious that language is not involved in this wonder. Although nonverbal communication is a preeminent channel in the transmission of information, its impact is frequently overlooked as an explanatory model of interactions.

The statistics surrounding the tragedy of suicide have already been presented. There is no disputing how disheartening it is to see suicide rates steadily increase. Project 2025 has been initiated to reduce the annual suicide rate by 20 percent by 2025. The focus of the American Foundation for Suicide Prevention includes four critical areas: firearms and suicide prevention, large health systems, emergency departments, and correction systems. These statistics make it imperative to consider multiple determinants influencing self-destructive behavior. To do this, we will have to think beyond strictly psychological or other intrapersonal motives (46).

In the late 1800s, Emile Durkheim, considered to be the father of sociology, studied suicide in France. It has been reported he made a wager predicting, one year in advance, the number of suicides that would occur in Paris, and he added to this prediction the number of suicides that would occur in different parts of the city. He could not divine who the particular individuals might be, but only the number of suicides. It is reported he won his bet. When asked to explain how he knew these results one year in advance, Durkheim replied that he had simply looked at the number of individuals who had committed suicide the year before. His classic work published in 1897, *Suicide: A Study in Sociology*, emphasized if we were to ever understand suicide, we had to look at the culture or social system and the existing mores from which people derive their conscience and moral support. Durkheim felt all ameliorative measures must be directed back to the question of social structure. He cautioned that an increase in suicide reflects a basic flaw in the social fabric; accordingly, increasing rates could not be halted through education alone.

After reviewing multiple influences that might precipitate suicides, including religious and family patterns, economic fluctuations, pathological states, etc., he still concluded that when social conditions fail to provide people with the necessary social goals and rules, then the most vulnerable will commit suicide. None of the factors and forces that shape our lives can explain suicide unless they are seen in the context of the fundamental structure of society. All ameliorative measures must ultimately be referred back to the question of social structure. He believed that a partial solution would consist in helping individuals perceive they are part of the social structure and its collective conscience. Durkheim believed that each society has a collective inclination toward suicide, which is fairly constant. All suicides were therefore not purely intrapersonal events. In other words, the suicide of individual members could only be understood as a reflection of the pressures within the society at large. Society has its quota of suicides, but the number varies according to the changes in the individual's particular social system. Suicide is an act of societal deviance and to better understand it, one must look at the communication within society.

Durkheim also believed crime, like suicide, has an important social function and, like suicide, it could not be eliminated. He further contended that the way in which society reacts to crime contributes to its overall health. Consequently, he felt the function of punishment is not the abolition of crime, which is impossible, but the reaffirmation of a social system's basic values. He did not believe every level of crime was healthy, but that deviance served an adaptive function and should be understood accordingly. Durkheim's is a functionalist approach to the understanding of deviance, of which both suicide and crime are expressions. Crime facilitates the unification of the social system in an attempt to solve and deal with this problem. Although his work preceded that of Freud, Durkheim felt that sociology as well as psychology had a role to play in understanding suicide (17).

As suggested, Durkheim's functionalist approach has not yet been integrated into our understanding of deviance. Just look at the suicide statistics previously presented in Chapter 3. As a concept, deviance does not simply refer to socially unacceptable behaviors. Geniuses would be considered deviants, because they deviate from the norm. Deviance is a term that describes individuals and behaviors that deviate from what is usually accepted within a given social system. Mass shootings are another example of extreme deviance. It follows that if we are to better understand this horror, beyond strictly individual motives, it may be beneficial to look at the communication influencing this behavior (19).

It may be difficult for the reader to consider that deviance may serve an adaptive function for society. It is not an intuitive approach to the understanding of self-destructive and violent acts. In our quest to better understand the human condition, we may have to become more practiced in considering alternative truths. An openness to thinking about this may actually simplify our understanding and reduce feeling of impotence in the face of societal ills.

In his excellent book *Wayward Puritans: A Study in the Sociology of Deviance*, Kai T. Erikson expanded Boas's functionalist ideas to explore the purpose of deviance. Deviance, according to Erikson, is a property conferred upon behavior by the community of individuals who come into contact with it. If deviant influences are perceived to disrupt the existing social order, pressures will be applied to eliminate this disturbance. For example, we have seen the reactions to marijuana legalization and same-sex marriages. Many members of our social system believed these behaviors would disrupt the existing social order. Consequently, in an attempt to reduce this disruption and maintain the status quo, the dangers of these behaviors were exaggerated.

Erikson analyzed three crime waves that occurred during the history of the Puritan settlement in 17th-century Massachusetts.

To the Puritans, the Bible served as the ultimate instrument of law, while ministers functioned as the final moral authority. A congregation, like a jury, was responsible for evaluating an individual's relationship to God. The first crime wave in the settlement was caused by the Antinomians—a name originally given to the heretics of Martin Luther's time. The group's deviations from accepted theory were considered to be disturbing to the existing order. To reduce this disrupting influence, many of the heretics were banished from the settlement.

The second crime wave arose from an influx of Quakers, who also challenged the Puritans' identity. The disruption initiated a wave of persecutions. Initially, Quaker housewives were arrested and their literature burned in the market place. The jailed women were stripped of their clothing and searched for marks of witchcraft. Male Quakers, for a first offense, had one of their ears cut off. They were then sent to the house of correction to work until they earned enough money to be banished. For the offence of continuing to practice and promote Quaker beliefs, their tongues were bored through with hot irons and beatings increased in severity. In time, the women were whipped and suffered the same sentence as the men. The Puritans actually shared many features in common with the Quakers, but the Puritans chose to publicize their differences only.

The Salem witch trails began in 1692, when several girls from the neighborhood began to spend their afternoons with a slave named Tituba, who was reputed to have dabbled in the magic arts. After a period of time, several of these girls would scream for no apparent reason, fall into convulsions, and sometimes drop to their hands and knees, barking like dogs. Their physician concluded the devil had come to Salem Village. This was the third crime wave. Hysteria ensued well beyond Salem Village, and these girls began to accuse people they had never seen of witchcraft. Their accusations were never questioned, but tests were administered to determine if the accused were really witches. Initially, they had to recite the Lord's Prayer and cure fits by touch—feats deemed impossible by witches. Their bodies were inspected for warts, moles, and scars through which the devil might have sucked blood. At least 19 people were executed, and three others died from different causes. Not one suspect brought before the court had ever been acquitted.

During the period from 1636 to 1682, the following were deemed categories of crimes against the Puritan church: disturbing the congregation, fornication (i.e., birth of a child too soon after a marriage), drunkenness, theft, assault, criticism of the government, and so on. The Puritans justified their merciless punishments by saying, "It makes no difference how severely the judge treats him, because all the suffering and hardships in this world would be nothing compared to the torments of an eternity in hell (18).

After a systematic analysis of all the available data about the three crime waves, Erikson drew conclusions in agreement with those of Boas. Deviance, if controlled, is a condition for preserving the stability of the society. Society requires its quota of deviants! If we look at crime rates, we will find they are stable over time. While the type of deviance may change, the number of deviants does not (8). This is similar to the views presented earlier about the constancy of suicide.

Today, we are understandably concerned by the proliferation of gun violence. What are the motives, and why should mass shootings have become so ubiquitous? Erikson points to the excessive coverage of school shootings on television and in newspapers. He wonders if this repetitive mode of inundating us is a replacement for and analogous to the same kind of mass information as social visits to the local prison or public hangings centuries ago. Is it possible that these sources of information are in part responsible for perpetuating the deviance they ostensibly discourage? I personally believe there is some truth in it. The murderer invariably knows the value of life but, for some, their motive might be to kill because it offends the most important value of the group. Through the excessive bombardment by television, a kind of credit is being stored in the deviant's perverted mental bank account that must be eventually spent.

I am suggesting a more tempered and judicious amount in the quantity of reporting and in the overwhelming publicizing of these crimes to help reduce the incidence of mass killings. This does not in any way negate the need for better identification of and treatment for the severely mentally ill, but sickness cannot be the only motive we search for when we try to understand such horrific deviance.

We have already touched upon the role of isolation and aggression. How many of the perpetrators of violence perceive themselves as isolated, apart from the existing social order. The impact and influence of prolonged psychological isolation and its relationship to deviance cries for investigation. This suggestion takes on a particular importance when we look at the scant research on gun deaths.

Every year, nearly 30,000 Americans die from gunshots. Yet US law has limited federal spending for gun violence research. It was recently reported that between January 1, 2009 and May 2018, there were 288 school shootings. This is 57 times higher than six G7 countries combined (52). However, according to the Centers for Disease Control and Prevention, between 2004 and 2015 only $22 million went into gun violence research. If gun violence were funded at a level proportional to the number of deaths it causes, the amount should have been $1.4 billion. Research on gun violence received less than one percent of the research funding that goes into research on sepsis, though both kill around the same number of Americans each year. Between 2004 and 2015, there were 1,738 research publications on gun violence compared to 43,477 publications on sepsis. Of the 49 months since January of 2014, only six have passed without at least one incidence of gun violence in a US school (52). I cannot overstate my belief that the media bears some responsibility for this communication of deviance. I am again asking for consideration of this position accompanied by a scientific evaluation from unbiased investigators.

During WWII and the Cold War, Hollywood made propaganda films for the sole purpose of influencing our behavior. We hated our enemies, purchased war bonds, and zipped up our lips so we did not sink ships. Later, in schools we had meaningless retention drills to protect ourselves from communist nuclear bomb attacks. Yet, when Hollywood today is questioned about the relationship between extreme violence in their films and the prevalence of antisocial acts and moral decline, they deny any correlation. When it was to their advantage, they took credit for the effectiveness of their propaganda films. Today, there are financial incentives to deny any responsibility for the influence of their films on antisocial behaviors. It is true many other countries have violent films and video games. While we share this exposure, only the US has easy access to guns, something not found in other societies.

I therefore propose the following study in order to investigate the possible influence of media communication. Several days before New Year's Eve, the press announces to the public that due to new automotive safety features and increased punishments for driving while intoxicated, a significant reduction in automotive accidents and deaths is predicted. After the holiday, compare the number of accidents and fatal injuries with statistics from prior years. Warnings to drive safely have previously done little to change the dreadful data. Why not consider a change in communication?

When I first entered graduate school, I worked on skid row. This was an area of Philadelphia where derelicts and the homeless were known to congregate. My function was to find one of three hospitals to admit serious alcoholics for treatment. If the hospitals had no beds available, I would take my client to a small all-night movie theater where for one dollar the homeless could safely stay the night. The next morning, I would return to the filled theater, pick up my client, and spend the day with them until they could be hospitalized for treatment. I came to share the belief that society demanded its quota of deviants.

The preference to live one's life on the streets is an individual's right, but it is also an expression of deviance. This is not a value statement or a judgement of any kind. There will always be those for whom life on the streets has more appeal, despite attempts to provide an alternative way. I am suggesting if you wish to control for this type of deviance, set aside an area of the city where the homeless will be safe. The location should be known to offer shelter, food, clothes, and medical attention. Instead of trying to eliminate the problem, plan for it; it is endemic to our social system, as are other expressions of deviance. Have all the arrests for various crimes stopped crime? Since legal punishments do not appear to serve as a deterrent, we are obligated to consider deviant behavior as it is determined by patterns of communication within the existing social order. Only then will we be able to effect real change.

Another example of nonverbal communication is illustrated by an experience I had that was similar to one shared by Arthur Koestler. This prolific writer authored books on a variety of subjects, from capital punishment to human creativity. He was also a correspondent, an émigré, a journalist, a dedicated anti-fascist, and for a time a communist. In 1937, while reporting on the Spanish Civil War, he was imprisoned for three months because communists were known for their opposition to the Spanish dictator, Franco. He was placed in solitary confinement and threatened with execution. Koestler, looking for metaphysical comfort in his situation, remembered the novel *Buddenbrooks* by Thomas Mann. In this novel, one of the main characters, who knows he is about to die, "realizes that death is not final, merely a transition to another, impersonal kind of existence, a reunion with cosmic oneness."

Remembering this passage gave Koestler some degree of comfort and, as luck would have it, he was released from prison. He had never written a fan letter, but on the day after his release, he wrote to Thomas Mann and thanked him for the comfort that he had derived from that passage. Mann wrote back to Koestler and explained that he had not read the essay that had inspired his book *Buddenbrooks* since 1897 or 1898, as he had never wanted it to weaken its original strong impact on him. However, one afternoon, Mann felt a sudden urge to read the original essay, went to his library, and obtained it after nearly 40 years. At that very moment, there was a ring at his door and the mailman handed him Arthur Koestler's letter (31).

I knew that Koestler's last book, *Bricks to Babel,* was being printed. I ordered it from the publisher and impatiently waited for the book to arrive. Week after week, I looked for the book as soon as I arrived home from work. Finally, one late afternoon the book was there. I went into my bedroom, propped myself up, turned on the television for background noise, and excitedly started to read. Just as I began, I heard the news that Arthur Koestler and his wife were found dead in a probable suicide pact. That was on March 3, 1983, and I wrote the following notation in the flyleaf: "the desert seems to have reclaimed the oasis." Later, I learned in addition to Parkinson's, Koestler suffered from leukemia and was an advocate of the right to die with dignity.

I have no psychic gifts and am skeptical about telepathy. This experience does, however, seem to be more than just a coincidence. I believe, as suggested earlier when describing the Einstein-Podolsky-Rosen paradox, that influences from nonverbal communication causally determine events we experience. These influences happen in a manner not immediately obvious and in ways we have yet to fully understand. This, however, does not prevent us from considering the impact of this communication on our social and personal behaviors.

Before moving on, I would like to present some additional assumptions that guide my thinking and offer them to the reader for consideration. I firmly believe that doubt is the beginning of wisdom. During my lectures, I may ask for a definition of randomness. The answers typically range from, "events that have an equal probability of occurring" to "events lacking a definite plan, purpose, or pattern." These are correct, but I offer another definition: randomness may be the behavior of events for which we have not yet found an explanation. I define religion as the systematic organization of fact, and science as a systematic organization of doubt. A scientific fact may simply represent a consensus of opinion, where a choice has been made to look no further. This is why scientific conclusions must be questioned and subject to repeated verification.

Before moving any further, I ask that you complete a simple quiz. Your true or false answers can be read as reflecting the models of behavior you hold.

1. The marriage of cousins is practically certain to result in children of inferior intelligence.

2. Long slender hands indicate an artistic temperament.

3. Adults sometimes become feebleminded from overstudy.

4. Emotional expression in another person can be judged more accurately from the eyes than from the mouth.

5. If you stare at a person's back, you can make him turn around. This is a form of telepathy.

6. Especially intelligent children are likely to be weak and physically retarded.

These statements have been proven to be false.

As we review the work of Rupert Sheldrake, please keep in mind what constitutes real science. Rupert Sheldrake is an English biologist and biochemist, an author and parapsychologist, who studies telepathy, precognition, psychokinesis, and other forms of ESP. As a biologist, he investigated morphogenetic fields, a concept central to biology and medicine. These fields are actually information bearing global patterns in chemoelectrical properties that guide our growth and form (44).

Sheldrake extends this concept to propose a new kind of evolutionary field. He assumes that the more patterns of development are repeated, the more probable it is that they will be followed again. He postulates these fields are the reason that habits of species are built up, maintained, and inherited. Remember Einstein's action at a distance, where subatomic particles interact with one another no matter how distant they may be. Sheldrake extrapolates these interactions to posit a process he calls morphic resonance—the influence of like upon like through space and time. For example, he suggests that penicillin crystallizes the way it does because it has crystallized that way before, and the information about crystallization has been passed onto future penicillin crystals regardless of the location where the penicillin is being produced. The same would be true if a scientist developed a new crystal after an extensive period of research and development. Sheldrake's suggestion is that when the hypothetical crystal were to be manufactured, it would take far less time because the chemicals involved had learned how to crystalize from the very first crystallization.

Sheldrake used the example of the tit study I presented earlier to suggest that telepathy might be an explanation for the cream-stealing habits of the birds. Another study employed to support his theory occurred between two counties in rural England. Both villages received their daily newspaper at the same time, and it was the habit of many residents to do the crossword puzzles. Sheldrake first measured the time it took members of both counties to solve the puzzles. He claimed the times were identical. Sheldrake then arranged for one county to receive the paper before the second county. He measured the time it took the members of the first county to solve the puzzle and compared it to the time required for those in the second county to solve the puzzle. Sheldrake found it now took less time for those in the second county to solve the identical puzzles. He concluded that the solutions of the puzzles were communicated from the first county to the second county, enabling the readers in the latter county to solve the puzzles more quickly. Sheldrake postulated that the communication between the members of the two counties occurred through his morphogenetic fields. His understanding of morphogenetic fields is based on his belief that morphic fields operate in social groups and are capable of connecting members of one group to other groups, even if they are miles apart. To Sheldrake, this quality of connectivity helps to explain what is sometimes called telepathy.

Sheldrake also inferred that if he divided a particular species of rats into two groups and taught one group in England how to learn a maze, the other group in America would learn the identical maze much quicker. Again, the knowledge would be transmitted across time and space through morphic resonance. He strongly believes that dogs have telepathic abilities, as do many other species of animals. He has observed, as others have, that dogs seem to anticipate the arrival of their owner. He has also explored the phenomenon of being stared at and a purportedly common form of telepathy that occurs with the telephone. He reports that more than 80 percent of the population say they have thought of someone for no apparent reason who then called or who was known to be calling before the conversation began.

He believes that morphic resonance is the basis of memory in nature. This concept suggests there are mysterious telepathy-type interactions between organisms and collective memories passed on within species. Morphic resonance implies that systems such as termite colonies, pigeons, plants, and even insulin molecules inherit a collective memory from previous things of their kind. This inheritance is said to be responsible for the telepathy-type interactions between living and nonliving matter (44).

There is little doubt that some of what Sheldrake presents we may ourselves have experienced. His theories can be philosophically interesting and seductive, but this does not necessarily make them scientific (40). Since doubt is the beginning of wisdom, one's first question might be: have Sheldrake's examples been subjected to experimental verification by others? In his case, the answer is no. Has his material been published in peer review journals? The answer appears to be the same, no. A critical question is, how do we measure morphic resonance? Is this concept consistent with what is known about genetics and embryology? This does not appear to be the case (45).

Science is self-correcting. The scientific method, ideally, is nondogmatic and hypotheses that are inconsistent with the observed data are rejected. Presently, there is a lack of evidence for Sheldrake's assumptions and we must conclude, until proven otherwise, that his science is pseudoscience. His theories were presented to illustrate that you should not be hesitant to use a rigorous scientific approach to challenge and question theories or beliefs, even though they may be advanced by so-called experts. You have the right and even the obligation to see and evaluate the beliefs of others according to your perspective, your models, and your thoughts. The strength and the growth of most disciplines reside in a navigation of differences, not an assertion of the need for consensus.

Dr. Steven Strogatz is a well-renowned professor of applied mathematics, presently at Cornell University. He uses math to explain our world through its application to physics, biology, and the social sciences. His work is well respected and presented in a passionate, scientific manner as he endeavors to communicate the value of mathematics to the public.

In 1995, Strogatz was influenced by two biologists David Welsh and Steve Reppert at Massachusetts General Hospital. They discovered that our brains contain a population of oscillators, which distribute natural frequencies that pull one another into synchrony. These oscillators are the cells of our circadian pacemaker, our internal chronometer keeping us in sync with the world around us. It is important to note that when groups oscillate together, it becomes more powerful than a single individual's oscillation. This is the science of sync (47).

It is believed this is the mechanism behind the syncing of menstrual cycles in females who often spend time together. This does not negate the unconscious pushing and pulling on one another's cycle that is also being mediated by pheromones. The understanding of this behavior is not yet clear, but group oscillation appears to have some explanatory validity.

Coupled oscillators facilitate things that cycle automatically. That is, they repeat themselves over and over again at regular time intervals. For example, fireflies tend to flash in a synchronous unison. Even if individual fireflies are separated from the others, they will continue to flash to a previously established steady beat. Each firefly contains an oscillator, the timing of which adjusts automatically in response to the flashes of other fireflies. Most of us have heard the crickets who seem to chirp in unison as well.

If infants are in sync, their sleep and feeding patterns are predictable. However, if their patterns are out of sync, the parents will be the first to know. Adolescents who prefer to stay up late and sleep in have their internal clocks set differently than when they were younger. The same is true for the elderly, who may wake up early in the morning and, no matter how tired, cannot fall back to sleep. They are felt to be out of sync. Previously, changes in lighting were suggested to help with the subject of sleep-arousal imbalance. Such modifications return us to the idea of an adaptive sync.

Additional problems are seemingly created when people have to alternate their working hours between day and night shifts. Medical and psychological problems plague many of these individuals. Strogatz points out the industrial accidents at Chernobyl and Three Mile Island both occurred between midnight and 4AM. Synchrony also regulates the relationship between various organs in our bodies. Ultimately, synchrony informs many of the interactions between ourselves and the world. Under normal circumstances, we are synchronized to a 24-hour day, driven mainly by sunrises and sunsets.

An interesting finding is the propensity for REM sleep to be synchronized to the body temperature cycle and not to sleep itself. REM sleep is most likely to occur just after the temperature cycle of the body is the coldest. The brain doesn't care whether it is the end or the start of sleep. However, in the normal 24-hour circadian phase, REM sleep occurs when most people wake up because it is the time when body temperature tends to be coldest (47).

We have all experienced group synchronization in one form or another. Consider the experience of being at a party when all of a sudden everyone stops talking. Another example is the reaction of a crowd at a musical concert, particularly their applause. Watch and hear the venom spew from the mouths of the marching neo-Nazis and the reaction of those opposing their intrinsic evil. Many will remember the hysteria of the McCarthy era when the mantra was "better dead than red."

Sync has offered us insights ranging from cardiac arrhythmias to sleep cycles. It is grounded in excellent science and rigorous mathematics, and has helped describe a wide range of cooperative behaviors in living and nonliving matter. We have only covered a small sample of the contributions of Dr. Strogatz and his colleagues who, through sync, revealed the hidden but beautiful order that governs the rhythms of nature as well as the rhythms within us. Group synchronization is an option to help us in our understanding of human behavior, both at the biological and the psychological level. It is also another example of the power of nonverbal communication.

When my son was in middle school, he had to complete a science project in class for the competitive science fair. He chose to investigate how playing Nintendo affected the capacity for attention and concentration in students. At that time, Nintendo was a popular gaming system and dominated the market. In a reasonably controlled study, my son administered pre-tests of attention and concentration. After the subjects played Nintendo, post-tests were administered. The results revealed that watching Nintendo had a negative effect on a student's ability to voluntary impose directed attention and concentration. It appeared those who played the game had their attention determined by the action, movement, and sounds from the TV screen. When these potent stimuli were absent, they had difficulties exhibiting self-imposed attention and concentration on the tasks. It was concluded from this limited study that watching Nintendo could have a negative effect on and interfere with self-directed attention and concentration. Nintendo eventually put a disclaimer on their game boxes, unrelated to this study, indicating that playing the game for a protracted period of time could cause seizures. This type of photosensitive epilepsy, rare at the time, has become more common as television and video games have gained in prominence. The disorder is believed to be related to dysfunction in synchronization; the flickering of the screen causes the neurons in the brain to misfire in lockstep and produce a seizure. This is a case where a fast, periodic signal arising in the external environment has an impact on human biology. Hopefully, environmental factors and their influence on our behavior will be considered with the same level of engagement as the other models presented above.

CONCLUSION

It takes courage, knowledge, and self-discipline to examine belief systems in others as well as oneself and move toward different understandings of behavior. Remember the question I posed to the administrator at the outset of the book: "Did you ever think the reason no scissors were missing is because I did not expect them to be?" I now honestly believe the reason none were taken is because I communicated a sincere trust in those patients. They perceived that it never entered my mind to think otherwise. If I did not think it, why should they? Had I acted differently and cautioned them to return the scissors, would the outcome have been different?

We have seen in the past as well as in the present how many individuals resist considering alternative models and refuse to change beliefs and behavior despite evidence to the contrary. This resistance seems ubiquitous and self-correction appears to be elusive, even to the best of us. More often than not, it is because we have been programed by our life experiences, our education, and the social system within which we reside. It is not an easy task to open to alternative ways of perceiving and questioning, even if it offers the potential for greater truths.

For a number of years, I supervised a child abuse program in a large section of Philadelphia. I sent one of my five family workers to evaluate a woman who was living with her four children in a two-room apartment. It was winter, and her only source of heat was a gas range located in a small kitchen next to the single room where she and her children resided. After this particular family worker returned from her evaluation, she was ready to have the Department of Human Services place the children into foster care. Instead of acting on her recommendation, I asked another one of my family workers to revisit the same family and give me her opinion of the situation.

When this worker returned, she did not see chaos but saw a mother who had implemented an impressive system under difficult circumstances. Each child had their specified turn to wash, dress, eat, and get ready for school. Two workers, two opposing views. Here was a mother who was making the best out of difficult circumstances. It would have been a dreadful mistake to remove her children. The appropriate thing to do was to provide adequate heat and locate a larger apartment.

One of the more obvious and influential models we hold is about aging. There is little doubt that thanks to modern medicine, improved nutrition, and other social factors, we are living longer. Many of the elderly are likely to remain reasonably active and involved well into their 70s and even their 80s. It is predicted that by the year 2020, when the baby boomer children are old, one out of every five of the population will be in their retirement years.

In the early part of the last century, the majority of those over age 65 lived with a child. The developers during this period continued to act on the belief that the elderly preferred contact with other generations. In 1960, this model changed and choices for the elderly increased. The impetus for this shift came from Del Webb, an Arizona real estate developer who popularized the term "retirement community." He built Sun City, a community in Phoenix that was the first to limit its residents to retirees. Webb held a different view, and Sun City reflected his vision of how people would spend their leisure years. There was a golf course, a shopping arcade, and a recreation center. Living with the family decreased and what emerged was a respect for the independent self (20). The concept of Sun City was developed with the hope of giving the elderly an opportunity to share experiences with their peers in a way that cultivated and respected their independence.

Aging is not merely about the passage of time, but also speaks to the number of significant social events. Our children grow up, move, and have families of their own. We retire and unfortunately may lose a spouse or partner. This often leads to boredom, loneliness, and sense of helplessness about it all. These changes are the reason for the creation of full-life facilities, which provide living arrangements for those who are still independent as well as others who require assisted living or full-time supervised nursing care.

For the past 14 years, I have functioned as a clinical neuropsychologist in just such a facility. During my time there, I have observed various forms of collective behavior that can partly be explained by group sync. A common example is the endless commentary about the food quality. No matter how hard the chefs prepare, present, and vary the menus, the next day they'll be met with a variety of complaints. What I find interesting is that these complaints do not have their basis in individuals, but in the dynamics of the group. This is understandable, as for many the highlights of the day are the meals; they are an occasion for people to come together.

I have also noticed that resident meetings are anticipated with indifference or disdain. Yet at the end of the meetings, I always hear thunderous applause. There is no doubt in my mind that the pull of nonverbal communication, perhaps synchrony, is responsible for this clapping. Often when I asked a resident, "How was the meeting?" invariably the answers sound the same: "no value," "same old stuff," "nothing changes." If one did not ask, one might infer something quite different from the applause. It would be easy to dismiss the above two examples as expected behavior. This assumption, while correct, would overlook that normal behavior is influenced by communication within the social milieu.

As I mentioned in Chapter 2, scientific advances have turned the process of aging and dying into medical experiences to be managed by health care professionals. Consequently, the management of advanced aging and dying has shifted to hospitals and nursing facilities. We have discussed these thoughts along with some of the strengths and limitations of the medical model. When working with the elderly, it is essential to become aware of the side effects of medication. Ninety percent of those over age 65 suffer from side effects that are often misdiagnosed as another illness. As a result, they are given additional medication for the new symptoms. Any symptoms in an elderly patient should be considered a possible side effect until proven otherwise (35).

I will be interested to see the future of the placebo in medical practice along with the recognition of the merits of hands-on phenomena. I believe it would greatly benefit the practice of medicine if more physicians integrated the psychogenic and sociogenic models of understanding human behavior.

For many elderly, there is not the slightest chance of medical intervention being of benefit. I have heard good medical practitioners softly say, "What do you expect, you are 90." Although medicine may not be able to repair the body, there is no reason why a person with anxiety and depression due to aging should be treated differently when seeking a medical examination. A 94-year-old individual has the right, when possible, to be free of pain and anxiety about their future.

It is also important to appreciate that these individuals are cut off from all the things that mattered to them in life. They may be in a nursing home, a medical center, or an ICU; however kindly they are treated, it tends to come from strangers. Have the number of geriatricians increased to deal with the increases in life span? I hope so. Taking care of the elderly is not always easy, as they may require more time to treat, have a litany of complaints, and ask questions for which there are no answers. Their problems cannot be fixed but still have to be understood and managed. If we wish to improve the quality of life for older individuals, then we must support their dignity, especially when they have reached the limit of life. At this stage, efforts should be directed to decrease incontinence, manage confusion, and help family members cope with devastating illnesses like Alzheimer's.

We touched upon the subject of death in Chapter 2. Now, however, we can understand a few observations in light of sync. I have observed a tendency for residents to pass away almost at the same time. When I would come to work, after a weekend off, my first stop was to read the death announcements. I observed that most were multiple deaths and that residents seemed to pass at similar times. Perhaps, the time and permission to die was being communicated to others. A unique sensitivity is communicated in the messages of sympathy from the residents, even if they did not know the deceased. There are, of course, multiple reasons for this; after all, they are members of the same living community as well as the community of humankind.

As previously mentioned, there appears to be a nonverbal communication of life and death that cries to be understood. One possibility is that evolution may have supported this form of communication. We have known for over 30 years that our adrenal glands and liver cells can display circadian rhythms of their own. This now appears to be true of heart and kidney cells as well. As with the communication of pain, is it not unreasonable to hypothesize that, like sync, the rhythms of individuals may also influence our living and dying (47)?

Twenty-two studies of older people published in *Psychology and Aging* found that negative age-related stereotypes caused short-term impairment in memory and cognition. Even minor differentiating gestures like speaking slowly or patronizing senior citizens could be hurtful. Very recently, a Yale University study looked at the impact of positive attitudes on the tendency to develop dementia. Their study involved 4,765 people, average age of 72, who were free of dementia. Twenty-five percent carried the APOE4 genotype, which increases the risk of developing dementia. The study lasted four years, and the results suggested that positive attitudes toward aging reduced the risk of dementia, even in the APOE4 carriers. We know that attitudes about aging are communicated and shaped by our culture as well as our life experiences. The researchers suggest positive attitudes may act as a buffer against stress and even affect the causal pathways by which the APOE4 gene expresses itself. It was suggested that health care providers try to identify those elderly with negative attitudes toward aging and encourage more positive attitudes to possibly improve cognitive health. This is but another example of how the communication within our social system influences behavior.

I have on my bookshelf a past bestseller *Final Exit: The Practicalities of Self-Deliverance and Assisted Suicide for the Dying*. It reflects the belief that the medical profession is remiss when they refuse the dying self-deliverance. The book provides dying people guidance on how to end their lives when their suffering became unbearable (29).

At the same time, I also keep a copy of the poem "Do not go gentle into that good night" by Dylan Thomas on my computer. The first stanza is as follows:

Do not go gentle into that good night

Old age should burn and rave at close of day;

Rage, rage against the dying of the light (48).

Which model of death and dying do you hold? Is death the ultimate enemy, or is death tantamount to intrinsic dignity? We know what Arthur Koestler believed. Sometimes, the suffering at the end of life is unavoidable and unbearable. Helping people end their misery may be appropriate. However, in every case, our beliefs determine how we interact and influence the elderly. If we are privileged to work with the terminally or severely ill, will it be in the form of assisted living or assisted dying?

Those of us who work or aspire to work in medicine and the helping professions must be aware that the family of a patient may become captured by the disease from which the patient suffers. They are held by commitments, love, obligations, and even guilt. Relatives may become as isolated as the patient, which has the potential to bring out long-standing family issues. The stress in a relative or caregiver may be communicated back to the patient, which sometimes has the effect of exacerbating the illness.

In my introduction, I discussed the downside of holding entrenched assumptions about the behavior of others. Dr. Drew's story is a prime example of how vital it is for all of us to become aware of the models determining our behavior. I have been accused of being an idealist. I am, but I do not equate idealism and naiveté. There will always be people who have a need to hate. However, those of us who strive to remove the scales from our eyes will be more effective and satisfied in our personal and professional lives.

Experience has taught me that far too many individuals suffer from what I call personal paranoia. There really is no such illness. It is just an expression I use to describe the feeling and belief that

"I am nothing." It is impossible for anyone to be nothing. Each and every individual has an impact on the rest of us in ways we may never appreciate. I hope by now I have given expression to the realization that to live is to affect others. For me, there is beauty in knowing we are all interrelated and perhaps even created from the same stardust.

My father loved to grow things. If he had two square inches of soil, he would plant something. My dad had grown a gardenia plant in an oversized pot. For as long as I can remember, when the flower bloomed, the aroma from the gardenia filled our home with its delightful fragrance. As my parents aged, they moved to a tiny apartment with a small outdoor balcony. The gardenia plant went with them. When my dad sat on the balcony to read the newspaper, the plant was beside him. Year after year, the plant thrived. He never spoke to the plant, but he tended to it with regularity. The day of my father's funeral, I felt an obligation to go to my parent's apartment to water the gardenia plant. As I arrived at the balcony where the plant sat, I was stunned to see it had died more than likely at the same time as my father.

It would help if professionals tried to better understand the role of nonverbal communication. Will the media ever consider they may have a role in contributing to the violence plaguing our society? I can only hope they heed it as one of the possible influences in order to help us understand the motives of the perpetrators so that we may increase our preventive efforts.

When I was an undergraduate in Temple University in Philadelphia, the Vietnam War was being fought overseas and at home on campuses throughout the country. I was part of the protests and would often be the first speaker at our rallies. I always tried to present an even-handed, rational approach to our position. There were usually thousands of students gathered for these events in the center of our campus. My involvement stopped when the rhetoric of subsequent speakers became confrontational and violent. Students took over buildings and stopped classes. There was no way to control the groupthink. It was as though thousands had become infected and were simply seduced by the fervor of the crowd. Several faculty members who knew me asked for my help in getting students out of the occupied buildings. Students commandeered a 10-story building having no idea what their next move would be. I was sent in to tell them the faculty would bring lunch if, after eating, the group agreed to leave the site. It worked because the group was glad to leave. Eventually, I witnessed the violence increase over issues that went well beyond the war. Several Ph.D. students were asked to leave school and deported to their homes in Canada. Today, I believe I was witness to an example of sync, coupled with verbal and nonverbal communications. The result was extreme and pervasive groupthink. These rallies seemed like they had a life of their own and many of us responded to the clarion call. At the extremes, was this behavior any different from those groups that hate because of differences in religion or nationality?

One day, while classes were in session, an African American student ran into the room and shouted, "Martin Luther King had been shot and killed." This happened throughout the campus, and the classrooms emptied out while thousands congregated in the area where rallies were held. There were no threats, just pacing that communicated an overwhelming sense of loss, frustration, disgust, helplessness, and most of all fear. The assassination of President Kennedy was still fresh in our minds and now another horrible killing. An eerie silence fell over the crowd, amplifying the fear. Crying young women would ask strangers to escort them to their cars. The fear caused the hair on the back of one's neck to stand up, and yet there were no outbursts. We all shared in this fear which, at times, bordered on terror. Without any signal, the crowd eventually dispersed leaving each of us to our private confusion. This was truly a communication unlike anything I experienced before or since.

Before the atomic bomb was dropped, we had to live with the prospect of our death as individuals. We now live before the horizon of our extinction as a species. We may not think about it consciously until we hear the saber rattling from North Korea as well as our own country. The acceptance of this possibility mirrors the acknowledgement of the ideas of Aristarchus, the Copernicans, Einstein, and Semmelweis. It appears all ideas have to go through an incubation period before a new idea can take hold and alter behavior. It seems that once an idea or model is invented, it cannot be easily disinvented. This is perhaps part of the pathology of our species. We can travel to distant planets, but struggle to deal fairly with immigration. We have the most destructive weapons on the planet, but cannot pass legislation to keep us from killing one another. There are unlimited funds for automotive bailouts but scant support for research on suicide or public education.

There is the distinct possibility that the evolution of technology has outpaced our present ability to properly manage it. Telepsychology may be an example of this phenomenon. It does, however, provide opportunities for individuals without access to therapeutic resources to obtain the help they need. These services have increased over the past decade, and I wonder if critical nonverbal information may be lost when the client is not in the room with the counselor. If a client is phobic, for example, but is being counseled in the security and safety of their home through teleconferencing, is it not possible the symptoms may be communicated differently? While this approach may have some advantages, the question is whether telepsychology becomes another financial venture or a modern treatment approach.

In the face of the complexities of medical and psychological needs, there is a relatively recent push for the formation of science teams to bring about evidenced-based solutions through cross-disciplinary approaches. The goal is to synthesize and build upon the methods, insights, and theories from a range of relevant disciplines to deal with human problems. However, the success of these endeavors will ultimately depend on the willingness of each individual to hold alternative models of behavior. Unless this happens, we will not have effective collaboration, only a collection of well-intentioned individuals (26).

It is disheartening to think that what is called human progress is largely an intellectual affair with substantially less invested in morality. I have slowly, and sometimes painfully, learned that any suggestion made to ask individuals to alter their beliefs meets with emotional resistance. Some resistance is due to ignorance and prejudice, but it can also take the form of legitimate resentment about the intrusion of unfamiliar challenges and ideas. When researching or treating a problem, please try to be open instead of bound by the dividing lines of your discipline. As we do not feel the pull of a magnet on our skin, we are often unaware how our beliefs fix our thinking and acting. The real value in holding multiple models or views of causality is in knowing that you are asking the correct questions. Is the behavior or event medical or psychological, or is it influenced by the patterns of communication in the environment? In the realm of truth, as we have seen, there is no ultimate authority. There are facts, but it is the model you use to interpret the facts that brings you closer to the truth.

For myself, I feel a major purpose in life is to put up the best performance possible. Doing so brings a sense of satisfaction to my life. The triumph of any endeavor is not only a triumph of intelligence, it is a triumph of character and integrity. It is my firm belief we should all be offended by unmerited misery, and so I ask the reader to give some consideration to the evidence our journey has revealed. I have put my hopes on this by word and example.

Selected Bibliography

1-Aboraya, Ahmed, M.D., et. al. (2018). "The Reliability of Psychiatric Diagnosis Revisited." *Psychiatry* 3 (2006): 41-50. Received from: http://www.ncbi.nim.nih.gov/pmc/articles/PMC2990547/.

2-Benson, Herbert (1975). *The Relaxation Response.* New York, N.Y. Harper Collins.

3-Birdwhistell, Ray, L. (1972). *Kinesics and Context: Essays on Body Motion Communication.* New York, N.Y: Ballantine Books, Inc.

4-______(1968). Communication Without Words. *Encyclopedia Des Sciences De L' Homme*, (5)157–166.

5-_______(1966). Human Communications and Human Potentialities, Springfield, Ill.: Charles C. Thomas. 309–322.

6-______(1974). *Lecture Notes,* University of Pennsylvania: Philadelphia, PA.

7-______ (2018). *Ray Birdwhistell.* Received from https://en.wikipedia.org/wiki/Ray_Birdwhistell.

8-Cahnman, Werner, J. "Book Reviews—Wayward Puritans." *Journal of the History of the Behavioral Sciences* 6 (1970): 367–368. Received from https://onlinelibrary.wiley.com/doi/abs/10.1002/1520-6696%28197010%296%3A4%3C367%3A%3AAID-JHBS2300060412%3E3.0.CO%3B2-3.

9-Carpenter, Siri (2012, September) Use of Probiotics. *Psychology Monitor.* 51–55.

10-Carrol, Aaron, E. (2018). *Do Antidepressants Work?* Received from https://www.nytimes.com/2018/03/12/upshot/do-antidepressants-work.html.

11-Carter Codell, K. and Barbara R. Carter (2008) *Childbed Fever—A Scientific Biography of Ignaz Semmelweis.* New Brunswick, New Jersey. Transaction Publishers.

12-Cho, Z.H., Wonk, E.K. and J. Fallon (2001). *Neuro Acupuncture.* University of California, Irvine, CA. 67–69.

13-(2018). *Contemporary Reaction to Ingaz Semmelweis.* Received from https://en.wikipedia.org/wiki/Contemporary_reaction_to_Ignaz_Semmelweis. 1–7.

14-Cooper, I.S., M.D (1981). *Vital Probe.* New York, N.Y: W.W. Norton & Company, Inc. 260–264.

15-(2018). *Couvade syndrome.* Received from https://en.wikipedia.org/wiki/ Couvade_syndrome.

16-Drew, Charles (2011). *Great Black Heroes.* Received from http://www.greatblackheroes.com/science/Charles-drew.

17-Durkheim, Emile (1951). *Suicide—A Study in Sociology.* Toronto, Ontario: Collier-Macmillian Canada, Ltd. 13–17, 189, 307.

18-Erikson, Kai, T. (1968). *Wayward Puritans, A study in the Sociology of Deviance.* New York, N.Y. John Wiley and Sons, Inc.

19-Functionalist Theories of Deviance. Received from https://www.d.umn.edu/~bmork/2306/Theories/BAMfunctionalism.htm.

20-Gawande, Atul. (2104). *Being Mortal, Medicine and What Matters in the End.* New York, N.Y. Henry Holt and Company, LLC. 1–20.

21-______(2007). *Better, A Surgeons Notes on Performance.* New York, N.Y. Henry Holt and Company, LLC. 1–24.

22-Ghose, Shohini. “The Einstein-Podolsky-Rosen Paradox and the Nature of Reality.” *La Physique Au Canada.* 65 (2009): 199.

23-Gravlee, Clarence. “Reanalysis of Franz Boas’ Immigrant Study. ” Received from http:www.gravlee.org/research/boas/.

24-Gupta, Sanja. (May 2018). CNN. Television Broadcast.

25-Halamka, John, D. (2011). “The Rise of Electronic Medicine.” *MIT Technology Review*, September 1, 2011. Received from https://www.technologyreview.com/s/425298/the-rise-of-electronic-medicine/. 1–8.

26-Hall, Kara, L. (May-June 2018). The Science of Team Science. *American Psychologist.*73 (4), 513.

27-Harlem, Steven (Unpublished paper; lecture notes). Temple University.

28-Harrington, Anne (2008). *The Cure Within, A History of Mind-Body Medicine.* New York, N.Y.,W.W. Norton & Company Ltd. 15–17, 64–65, 190–193.

29-Humphry, Derek (1991). *Final Exit.* New York, N.Y. Dell Publishing.

30-Katz-Sanger, Margot (2018). “Why is U.S. Health Care So Expensive?” Received from https://www.nytimes.com/2018/03/13/upshot/united-states-health-care-resembles-rest-of-world.html.

31-Koestler, Arthur (1980). *Bricks to Babel.* New York, N.Y. Random, House).

32-________(1963) *The Sleepwalkers—A History of Man's Changing Vision of the Universe.* New York, N.Y. Grosset & Dunlap. 536.

33-Kovacs, Lajos, et. al. (2014). *100 Chemical Myths, Misconceptions, Misunderstandings, Explanations.* Springer Cham. Heidelberg, New York, Dordrecht, London. 134–136.

34-Lama, Dalai and Desmond Tutu (2016). *The Book of Joy.* Avery, N.Y. (96).

35-Matteson, William (2016). Understanding Older Minds. *Health Ed.,* Eau Claire, WI.

36-"20 Medical Technology Advances: Medicine in the Future-Part 1." *The Medical Futurist,* July 14, 2016. Received from: https://medicalfuturist.com/20-potential-technological-advances-in-the-future-of-medicine-part-i.

37-Mendel, Gregor. (2018). Received from https://en.wikipedia.org/wiki/Gregor_ Mendel.

38-Muller, Richard, A. (2016). *The Physics of Time.* New York, N.Y. W.W. Norton & Company. 8–33.

39-Opioid Crisis. (May 2018) *The Kiplinger Letter.* Washington, DC. 1.

40-Pigliucci, Massimo (2010). *Nonsense on Stilts—How to Tell Science from Bunk*. Chicago. The University of Chicago Press. 1–14.

41-Relli, Carlo (2009). *The First Scientist—Anaximander and his Legacy*. Yardley, Pennsylvania, Westholme Publishing, LLC. 12–16.

42-Sacks, Oliver (2018). "Music and the Brain." Received from https://musicandmemory.org/music-brain-resources/music-and-the-brain/.

43-Sheldrake, Rupert (1994). *The Rebirth of Nature, Science and God*. Rochester, Vermont, Park Street Press.

44-_________(2018) *Rupert Sheldrake*. Received from https://Wikipedia.org/wiki/Rupert Sheldrake.

45-Strogatz, Steven (2003). *Sync—How Order Emerges From Chaos in the Universe, Nature and Daily Life*. New York, N.Y., Hyperion Books. 12–50.

46-(2018). Suicide Statistics. Received from American Foundation for Suicide Prevention. https://afsp.org/about-suicide/suicide-statistics/.

47-Thomas, Dylan. "Do not go gentle into that good night." Received from https://www.poets.org/node/44729.

48-Timimi, Sami (2018). "Does Psychiatry Actually Diagnose?" Interview by Eric R. Maisel Ph.D. *Psychology Today,* December 20, 2016. Received from https://www.psychologytoday.com/us/blog/rethinking-mental-health/201612/does-psychiatry-actually-diagnose.

49-Tomb, David, A, M.D. (1984). *Growing Old—A Handbook for You and Your Aging Parents.* New York, N.Y., Viking Penguin, Inc. 3–11.

50-*Understanding the* Opioid *Crisis.* (2018). Received from http://www.hhs.gov/opioids/about-the-epidemic.

51-(2018). US gun violence in six chilling statistics. Received from http://www.theweek.co.uk/91679/us-gun-violence-in-six-chilling-statistics. 1–11.

52-Weiss, Rick (November 28, 1995). *Is Nausea in Pregnancy Nature's Way of Protecting the Fetus From Toxins?* Received from https://www.washingtonpost.com/archive/lifestyle/wellness/1995/11/28/is-nausea-in-pregnancy-natures-way-of-protecting-the-fetus-from-toxins/387cd3c2-de3f-496a-96ac-0bc446733105/?utm_term=.8d65da330a62. 1–2.

53-Whitaker, Robert (2002). *Mad in America—Bad science, bad medicine and the enduring mistreatment of the mentally ill.* Cambridge, Mass. Perseus Books. 3–13, 41–63, 107–149, and 161–174.

54-__________(2005) "Anatomy of an Epidemic: Psychiatric Drugs and the Astonishing Rise of Mental Illness in America." *Ethical Human Psychology and Psychiatry*. 7 (2005). 23–35. Received from http://freedom-center.org/pdf/anatomy_of_epidemic_whitaker_psych_drugs.pdf.

55-Winerman, Lea. "Scant Research on Gun Deaths." *Monitor on Psychology,* April 2018.

48-Timimi, Sami (2018*)*. "Does Psychiatry Actually Diagnose?" Interview by Eric R. Maisel Ph.D. *Psychology Today,* December 20, 2016. Received from https://www.psychologytoday.com/us/blog/rethinking-mental-health/201612/does-psychiatry-actually-diagnose.

49-Tomb, David, A, M.D. (1984). *Growing Old—A Handbook for You and Your Aging Parents.* New York, N.Y., Viking Penguin, Inc. 3–11.

50-*Understanding the* Opioid *Crisis.* (2018). Received from http://www.hhs.gov/opioids/about-the-epidemic.

51-(2018). US gun violence in six chilling statistics. Received from http://www.theweek.co.uk/91679/us-gun-violence-in-six-chilling-statistics. 1–11.

52-Weiss, Rick (November 28, 1995). *Is Nausea in Pregnancy Nature's Way of Protecting the Fetus From Toxins?* Received from https://www.washingtonpost.com/archive/lifestyle/wellness/1995/11/28/is-nausea-in-pregnancy-natures-way-of-protecting-the-fetus-from-toxins/387cd3c2-de3f-496a-96ac-0bc446733105/?utm_term=.8d65da330a62. 1–2.

53-Whitaker, Robert (2002). *Mad in America—Bad science, bad medicine and the enduring mistreatment of the mentally ill.* Cambridge, Mass. Perseus Books. 3–13, 41–63, 107–149, and 161–174.

54-__________(2005) "Anatomy of an Epidemic: Psychiatric Drugs and the Astonishing Rise of Mental Illness in America." *Ethical Human Psychology and Psychiatry.* 7 (2005). 23–35. Received from http://freedom-center.org/pdf/anatomy_of_epidemic_whitaker_psych_drugs.pdf.

55-Winerman, Lea. "Scant Research on Gun Deaths." *Monitor on Psychology,* April 2018.